T0161979

THE
ANTI-INFLAMMATORY
Plan

Published by Welbeck Balance.
An imprint of Welbeck Publishing Group Limited
20 Mortimer Street
London W1T 3JW

Text © Anoushka Davy 2020
Recipes by Heather Thomas © Welbeck Non-Fiction Limited,
part of Welbeck Publishing Group Limited 2020

Design © Welbeck Non-Fiction Limited,
part of Welbeck Publishing Group Limited 2020

The right of Anoushka Davy to be identified as the author of this work
has been asserted by her in accordance with the Copyright, Designs
and Patents Act 1988.

All rights reserved. No part of this publication may be reproduced,
stored in a retrieval system, or transmitted in any form or by any means
(including electronic, mechanical, photocopying, recording, or
otherwise) without prior written permission from the publisher.

ISBN 978-1-85906-472-6

A CIP catalogue for this book is available from the British Library.

Printed in Spain

10 9 8 7 6 5 4 3 2 1

This book is not intended as a substitute for the medical advice of
physicians. Always consult health professionals in matters relating to
health and particularly in regards to any symptoms that may require
diagnosis or medical attention.

THE
ANTI-INFLAMMATORY
Plan

Prevent and reduce chronic inflammation to guard against ill health

ANOUSHKA DAVY

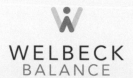

WELBECK
BALANCE

CONTENTS

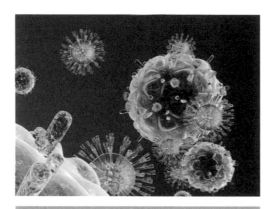 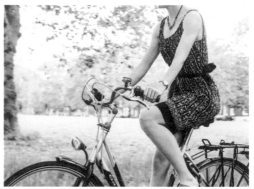

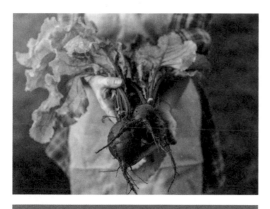

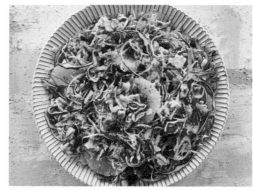

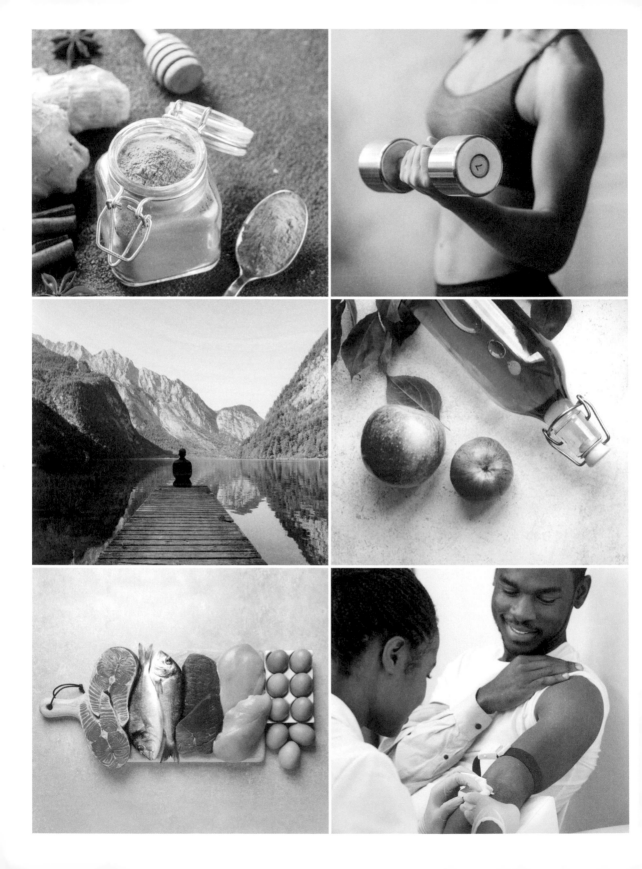

INTRODUCTION

There is an underlying process that connects and explains most, if not all, chronic disease. It explains heart attack, stroke, osteoporosis and cognitive decline. It connects seemingly disparate conditions such as asthma, eczema and fertility issues. It is also the process that lies at the heart of many ailments, such as aching limbs, stuffy noses and painful migraines. That process is inflammation.

Inflammation is fundamentally meant to be a helpful process, but as you will read in this book, there are many aspects of our diet and lifestyle that can trigger and perpetuate inflammation, sending it into overdrive. When inflammation is sustained over a long period of time, it can wreak havoc on your body and significantly increase your risk for developing various diseases including cancer, diabetes and heart disease. Inflammation can also cause you to age prematurely; it is now widely understood to be the main reason we age (so much so that it is now dubbed 'inflammaging'). More and more people are suffering from chronic inflammation at a younger age, and as a result experiencing poor health and a significantly reduced quality of life.

Targeting the underlying causes of inflammation, eating an anti-inflammatory diet and adjusting your lifestyle are the most powerful and effective ways to keep yourself well and prevent disease. In these pages you will discover the main causes of inflammation, including dietary, lifestyle and environmental triggers, and understand the most important changes you need to make to reverse and to prevent inflammation. This advice will help you to uncover the areas of your health that are fanning the flames of inflammation and need the most support and give you valuable tools to nurture your body and set you on the path to optimal health. In the last chapter, you will find a selection of 30 recipes, including breakfast, main meal, snack and dessert options. Each recipe has been carefully created to be fresh, delicious and packed full of anti-inflammatory ingredients. To your health!

Anoushka Davy

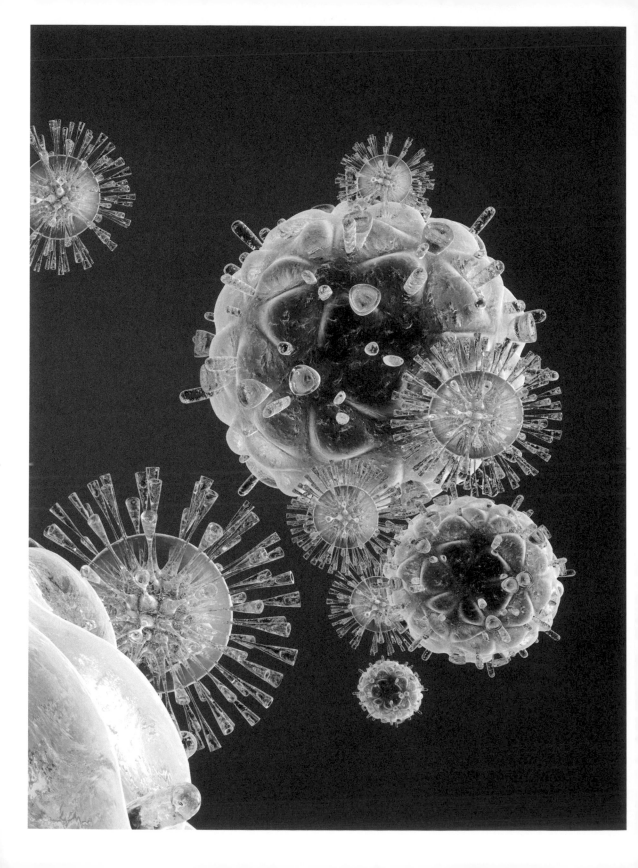

THE SCIENCE

In this chapter you will discover why the inflammatory response is such a vital part of keeping you healthy, the difference between acute and chronic inflammation and how long-term inflammation can increase your risk of developing chronic disease. The environmental, diet and lifestyle factors that cause chronic inflammation are explained and there is a quiz to help you identify which areas of your health need the most support to keep inflammation at bay.

WHAT IS INFLAMMATION?

Before we get into the details of why, when and how inflammation occurs, let's begin with a simple explanation of inflammation.

Inflammation is the body's way of responding to things that can cause harm, such as injury or infection. It is a complex process involving many different chemicals. The body initiates this process in an attempt to protect and heal itself.

When inflammation is helpful

While our planet is profoundly beautiful, it can also be dangerous. Our bodies are exposed to a multitude of harmful bacteria, viruses and toxic chemicals every day. The body has an impressive array of defence mechanisms to protect us from these dangers and inflammation is one of its most useful tools. An important biological function of our immune system, inflammation protects us from harm and keep us healthy.

Inflammation can stop infection, clear toxic substances and seal off and heal open wounds. You will know your body is responding with inflammation by spotting one of the five major signs of acute inflammation: redness, swelling, heat, pain and loss of function. Although these symptoms may be uncomfortable, they are essential to our survival. In fact, without inflammation, we would be dead pretty quickly – wounds would fester and infections would rapidly become life-threatening. Think of some common incidents – a paper cut, a bump on the knee, eating lukewarm seafood at a dodgy-looking buffet; in these situations the body instantly mounts an inflammatory response to rectify the situation and keep you safe. Your immune system works hard for you every day, responding to danger, helping you to heal and preventing minor issues from escalating into major threats.

Imagine your immune system as an army and inflammation as its weapon. Within an army, there are many different roles – sniper, demolitions expert, tank commander, and so on. This is much like the immune system, except the personnel are white blood cells, antibodies, histamine, complement proteins and messaging molecules called cytokines (which can either be pro-inflammatory or anti-inflammatory. These troops are stationed throughout your body, waiting on standby. After an initial stimulus, such as invasion of harmful bacteria, the troops are mobilized to launch an attack. White blood cells are usually first to the scene and can ambush in a variety of ways: some attack germs or damaged cells directly, some produce antibodies and some secrete inflammatory cytokines that ramp up the inflammatory process. Once the threat has been neutralized and there is no longer any danger, the troops will leave the area and balance will be restored. This process is called acute inflammation, which the body aims to resolve as quickly as possible to limit any collateral damage.

Five signs of inflammation

Inflammation can stop infection, clear toxic substances and seal off and heal open wounds. You will know your body is responding with inflammation by spotting one of the five major signs of acute inflammation.

- Redness
- Swelling
- Heat or fever
- Pain
- Loss of function

The inflammatory response

Inflammation occurs in response to infection, injury (a splinter in the skin, as here) or harmful toxins. It involves a complex sequence of biochemical events, which include the release of chemical messengers (such as histamine), a widening of blood vessels, increased blood flow and the movement of plasma and immune cells (such as neutrophils) to the site of the threat. Acute inflammation is characterized by the five cardinal signs (see above). Once the threat has been neutralized, the inflammatory response will resolve and normal functioning of the surrounding tissues can resume.

1. Cells near the injury site release chemical signals (histamine)

2. Capillary widens with increased blood flow

3. Migration of white blood cells (secreting pro-inflammatory cytokines) to the site of the injury to consume bacteria

4. Platelets move out of the capillary to seal the wound

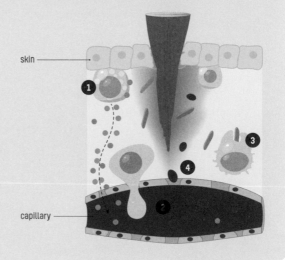

skin

capillary

Chronic inflammation: when things get out of control

Inflammation can be likened to fire – useful when small and controlled, but dangerous when uncontained.

After the immune system has dealt with an issue, inflammation should calm down, so physiologically things can return to normal. If the issue is not resolved, however, the small, helpful fire can become a raging, destructive force. When the immune system continues to fan the flames of inflammation in a misdirected attempt at healing, it can wreak havoc. This is what is known as chronic inflammation.

Chronic inflammation can damage your DNA, promote the build-up of dangerous plaque in your arteries and disrupt your brain function. It can damage tissues and create internal scarring. It can drive disease processes that increase your risk of developing chronic health conditions and slowly degrade your health.

Chronic inflammation underpins conditions such as heart disease, cancer and stroke; conditions that take millions of lives each year. It is also the driving force behind a plethora of common health issues that can seriously impact your quality of life, such as fatigue, headaches and weight-loss resistance. You won't find the answer to chronic inflammation in a pill or bottle, and while medication can help to reduce or alleviate symptoms, it won't address the reason inflammation started in the first place. The answer to resolving or preventing chronic inflammation lies in your hands, through the positive changes you can make to the way you eat, move and live, to help you feel better and brighter and dramatically change the trajectory of your health.

What starts as the tool to keep you healthy and protect you from harm, paradoxically becomes the very thing that threatens the foundations on which your health is built.

Chronic inflammation is linked to the development of several diseases and conditions, including:

- Alzheimer's
- Asthma
- Atherosclerosis
- Attention deficit hyperactivity disorder (ADHD)
- Autism
- Autoimmune conditions such as Hashimoto's thyroiditis and rheumatoid arthritis
- Cancer
- Chronic fatigue syndrome
- Dementia
- Depression
- Endometriosis
- Fertility issues
- Inflammatory bowel disease
- Irritable bowel syndrome (IBS)
- Obesity
- Polycystic ovary syndrome (PCOS)
- Skin issues such as eczema, psoriasis and acne
- Stroke
- Type 2 diabetes

Acute versus chronic inflammation

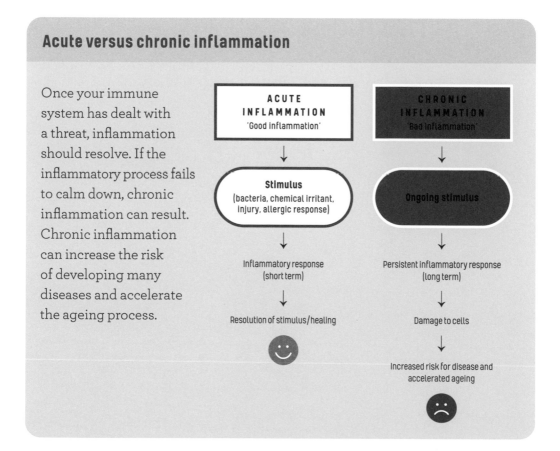

Once your immune system has dealt with a threat, inflammation should resolve. If the inflammatory process fails to calm down, chronic inflammation can result. Chronic inflammation can increase the risk of developing many diseases and accelerate the ageing process.

ACUTE INFLAMMATION
'Good inflammation'

↓

Stimulus
(bacteria, chemical irritant, injury, allergic response)

↓

Inflammatory response
(short term)

↓

Resolution of stimulus/healing

CHRONIC INFLAMMATION
'Bad inflammation'

↓

Ongoing stimulus

↓

Persistent inflammatory response
(long term)

↓

Damage to cells

↓

Increased risk for disease and accelerated ageing

HOW INFLAMMATION AFFECTS THE BODY

Here are some examples of how inflammation affects various parts of the body.

Cardiovascular system

Chronic inflammation is recognized as the main driving force behind the development of atherosclerosis. A sustained level of inflammation can encourage plaque formation and trigger blood clots, both of which can significantly increase the risk of heart attack and stroke.

Brain

The brain is separated from the immune system by the blood-brain barrier, a tightly packed layer of cells that lines the blood vessels to the brain. The brain does, however, have its own immune system, called the neuroimmune system, which protects the brain from foreign cells, toxic chemicals and infection. When the neuroimmune system responds to a harmful, stimulus, inflammation occurs in the brain and central nervous system. Ongoing inflammation can increase the risk of depression, anxiety and neurodegenerative diseases such as Parkinson's and Alzheimer's.

Muscle

Skeletal muscle is the most abundant tissue in the human body and cytokines (signalling molecules that stimulate or dampen an inflammatory response) play an important role in the synthesis and breakdown of muscle tissue. An excess of inflammatory cytokines, causing chronic inflammation, can result in muscle wastage. The balance can be skewed by many factors, especially age. Chronic inflammation is a key factor in the development of sarcopenia, an age-related degenerative condition characterized by loss of muscle mass, strength and function.

Bones

Osteoporosis, a condition in which bones become brittle, has been attributed to various hormonal, nutritional and metabolic factors, including vitamin D and calcium deficiency, low levels of sex hormones (such as low oestrogen in post-menopausal women), thyroid problems and a sedentary lifestyle. Research suggests that inflammation also exerts significant influence on bone regeneration. Certain pro-inflammatory cytokines have been implicated in the regulation of bone turnover and it is thought that chronic inflammation is a key risk factor for osteoporosis and other bone conditions.

Skin

The skin is an important first line of defence against harmful microbes and toxins. When the skin's immune system becomes overactive and chronic inflammation develops, various inflammatory skin diseases, such as psoriasis, rosacea and eczema, may develop.

Lungs

Chronic inflammation in the lung area can lead to breathing problems, and conditions, such as asthma and chronic obstructive lung disease. Chronic inflammation in the airways can be triggered by several factors, including cigarette smoke, air pollutants and imbalances in the lung microbiota.

Thyroid

Hashimoto's thyroiditis is the most common thyroid disorder, affecting millions of people globally. Hashimoto's is characterized by chronic inflammation of the thyroid gland. This leads to progressive destruction of thyroid tissue and results in an underactive thyroid. Chronic inflammation can also inhibit several genes involved in thyroid hormone metabolism, which can result in altered thyroid hormone production, such as decreased thyroxine (T4) and triiodothyronine (T3) and increased reverse T3, which can lead to an underactive thyroid (hypothyroidism).

Gut

The gut houses 70 per cent of the cells that make up our immune system, and plays a very important role in defending us from pathogens and toxins that we ingest on a daily basis. There are many factors that can trigger chronic inflammation in the gut, including intestinal permeability (also called leaky gut syndrome), food sensitivities and disruptions in the gut microbiota. Chronic inflammation of the gut can lead to the development of inflammatory bowel disease (ulcerative colitis and Crohn's disease).

Kidneys

Chronic inflammation is a hallmark feature of kidney disease. High levels of C-reactive protein, a marker of inflammation, in the bloodstream appear to accompany reduced renal function and chronic kidney disease (CKD), the most common form of kidney disease.

Reproductive system

Research indicates that chronic inflammation may be a key factor in reproductive dysfunction. Chronic inflammation can exacerbate conditions such as polycystic ovary syndrome and endometriosis. Inflammation affects many components needed for reproduction, and is a major cause of infertility in both men and women.

ROOT CAUSES OF INFLAMMATION

What causes our immune system to stay in battle mode? Why does something intended to help us cause such chaos?

Chronic inflammation occurs as a result of the immune system responding to a continual, unresolved threat. This prevents the completion of the healing process and allows inflammation to run riot. There are a multitude of different triggers that can cause the immune system to go into overdrive and cause chronic inflammation. These include:

- Diet

- Blood sugar issues and insulin resistance

- Stress

- Infection

- Gut issues

- Toxins

- Genes

- Lifestyle factors such as smoking, excess alcohol intake and lack of exercise

Diet

Food contains potent chemical messengers. Every bite you take can either send your body positive messages that inspire health and vitality, or send danger signals that trigger the immune system to respond with inflammation.

Modern diets are one of the main reasons we experience so much inflammation, and processed foods are the major culprits. These items are full of sugar, refined fats, preservatives, colourings and all sorts of weird and not so wonderful ingredients to enhance the flavour and prolong shelf life. The top three inflammatory foods are sugar, refined fats and oils and artificial sweeteners.

Sugar

Eating too much sugar is a sure-fire way to induce inflammation. Excess intake has been linked to insulin resistance, weight gain, tooth decay, damage to the gut lining and a reduction in the diversity of your gut bacteria, all of which can trigger and perpetuate a cycle of chronic inflammation.

Refined fats and oils

Fats are delicate and quickly become damaged when exposed to heat, light or chemicals. Consuming damaged, refined fats creates oxidative stress in the body. Oxidative stress can result in widespread inflammation and occurs when there is an imbalance between free radicals (unstable atoms that can damage cells) and antioxidants.

Refined oils are a mainstay of processed foods and often used in restaurant cooking. When reading a food label, you will know the product contains processed fats if you see words such as 'refined vegetable oil', 'hydrogenated', 'partially hydrogenated' or 'margarine'. You can also spot a refined oil if the label lists the oil but doesn't include the term 'extra virgin' or 'cold-pressed'.

Look out for industrial seed oils, which are highly inflammatory and bear no resemblance to natural fats. These include corn, soybean, rapeseed/canola, cottonseed, safflower and sunflower oil. These oils are exposed to extremely high temperatures, then processed with chemicals to improve the colour and taste.

Industrial seed oils have only been a part of our diet since the early 1900s and became widespread once companies became aware of their low cost and long shelf life. They have been cleverly marketed and their ability to cause harm has not received nearly as much attention as sugar. When you start reading labels and getting curious you will be shocked to see how much they have infiltrated our food supply.

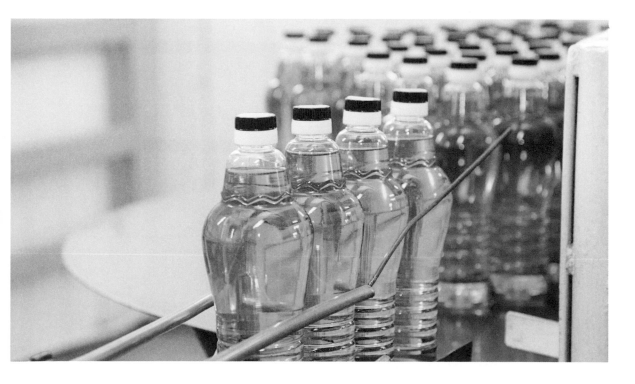

Artificial sweeteners

Used in many foods to improve taste, especially in those labelled 'diet' or 'light', artificial sweeteners include acesulfame, aspartame, neotame, saccharin and sucralose. Although they don't contain sugar, these ingredients can cause as much, if not more, metabolic dysfunction, which can lead to inflammation and increase your risk for conditions such as obesity, diabetes and cardiovascular disease.

Many people opt for products with artificial sweeteners to reduce their calorie intake, but this approach can backfire. One study, spanning seven years, found that regular consumption of artificially sweetened drinks doubled the risk of obesity[1]. Also of concern is the impact that sweeteners can have on our gut microbiota (the ecosystem of bacteria and other microbes that live in the gut). Studies have shown that the consumption of artificial sweeteners can negatively affect the composition and function of gut microbiota. This is important as imbalances in our gut microbiota can lead to inflammation.

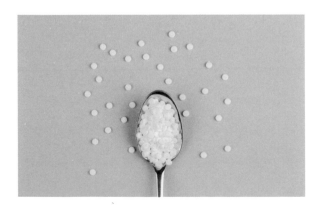

Blood sugar and insulin resistance

How well we balance our blood sugar levels plays a large role in our level of inflammation. Most people eat a diet that is high in the foods that drive up blood sugar levels. Our bodies hate having elevated blood sugar levels, and have sophisticated systems in place to maintain the right level. The complications of poorly managed diabetes – nerve damage, kidney failure and even limb amputation – indicate just how toxic raised blood sugar can be.

The main dietary factors that increase blood sugar levels are sugar and the over-consumption of simple or refined carbohydrates (such as white bread, chips, potato crisps, biscuits, many breakfast cereals, desserts, and so on), which break down into sugars. If simple carbohydrates and sugar take centre stage in your diet, this can lead to elevated blood sugar levels and, over time, insulin resistance. Insulin resistance can also be driven by stress and lack of exercise.

What is insulin resistance?

When you eat a meal containing carbohydrates, your blood sugar levels start to rise. In response to this, insulin, a hormone produced by the pancreas, is released. Insulin then travels through the bloodstream acting as a doorman, knocking on the door of your cells and telling them to open up and let in the sugars (glucose). Once insulin has done its job and the sugars have been taken up by your cells to be used as fuel or stored as fat, blood sugar levels fall back to normal.

If your blood sugar levels go too high too often, your cells can stop responding to insulin properly. Insulin will knock on the door, but the cells won't answer and glucose won't be able to get into the cell. This is called insulin resistance. Insulin resistance leads to chronically elevated blood sugar and symptoms such as fatigue and carbohydrate cravings because your cells lack an energy source. The pancreas responds to the high blood sugar levels by secreting more insulin, which in turn leads to chronically elevated insulin levels. Insulin resistance is one of the main drivers of chronic inflammation.

How well we balance our blood sugar levels plays a large role in our level of inflammation.

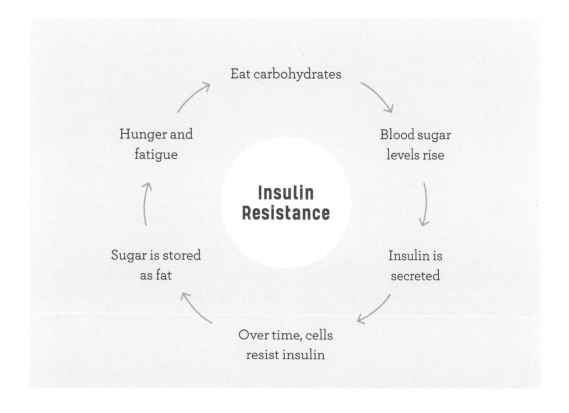

Infection

A lingering infection can be a big trigger for inflammation and can quietly fan the flames for months or even years. Some examples include dental infections, persistent viral infections, candida overgrowth, Lyme disease and its co-infections, sexually transmitted infections, such as chlamydia, parasites and many different types of harmful or opportunistic bacteria, fungi and mould that can get a foothold in the gut and other parts of the body. If there is an infectious cause behind chronic inflammation, tracking it down and treating it is essential to turning off the inflammatory response.

Dental infections can be particularly troublesome. There is a large body of research linking oral infection such as gum disease (periodontitis) with the initiation and progression of several conditions such as rheumatoid arthritis, cardiovascular disease and diabetes. This is because the infection spreads from the oral cavity to other parts of the body, triggering systemic inflammation. Root canals are also important to consider, as they can act as a reservoir for infection long after the root canal procedure has been completed. The lingering presence of bacteria in the root canal, as well as the harmful toxins these bacteria can produce, can be powerful drivers of inflammation.

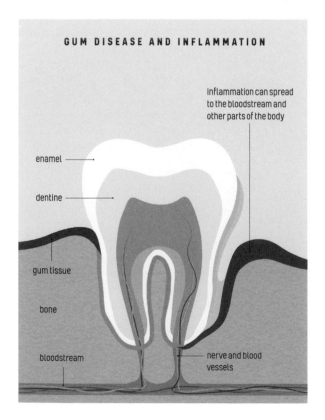

GUM DISEASE AND INFLAMMATION

inflammation can spread to the bloodstream and other parts of the body

enamel

dentine

gum tissue

bone

bloodstream

nerve and blood vessels

Stress

When stress dominates our lives and we lack the resources to cope, we are setting ourselves up for inflammation. The causes of stress are different for everyone. For one person, it may be a high-powered job combined with an intense exercise regime without adequate rest and nourishment as a counterbalance. For another, it may be a toxic relationship, money worries or loneliness. Stress causes inflammation by increasing the production of stress hormones and pro-inflammatory cytokines and by raising blood sugar levels and decreasing insulin sensitivity.

Gut issues

The gastrointestinal system is a marvel of biology. Your gut is able to take external matter, process it through a carefully orchestrated symphony of digestive processes, and end up with tiny molecules that can be used to power every cell. It is home to 70 per cent of your immune system and is in constant dialogue with your brain through the communication highway known as the vagus nerve. The microbiota in your gut comprise an incredible ecosystem of tens of trillions of microorganisms. It's a mutually symbiotic relationship – we give them a home, in exchange they do several important jobs, including keeping harmful microbes at bay and producing valuable nutrients such as short-chain fatty acids, B vitamins and vitamin K. They also synthesize neurotransmitters, such as serotonin, gamma aminobutyric acid (GABA) and dopamine, all of which play a key role in mood (who would have thought that bacteria could bring happiness ?!).

Our guts are under attack from poor diet, antibiotics, stress, over-use of certain drugs such as painkillers (especially non-steroidal anti-inflammatory drugs, or NSAIDs, such as ibuprofen), alcohol and smoking. These factors compromise our digestive function and significantly disrupt the health and diversity of our microbiota. Consequently, more people than ever are suffering from conditions such as acid reflux, irritable bowel syndrome and inflammatory bowel disease. Research has linked damage to the

THE ROLE OF DIET ON GUT MICROBIOTA

Your diet can alter the gut microbiota associated with inflammation. A diet high in fat and sugar decreases short-chain fatty acids (SCFAs) and antimicrobial peptides (AMPs), mucus production and protein junctions between cells in the intestinal wall.

Prebiotic and probiotic diets increase SCFAs, AMPs, mucus and tight protein junctions, and beneficial bacteria, such as lactobacillus and bifidobacterium, preventing such conditions as leaky gut and IBS.

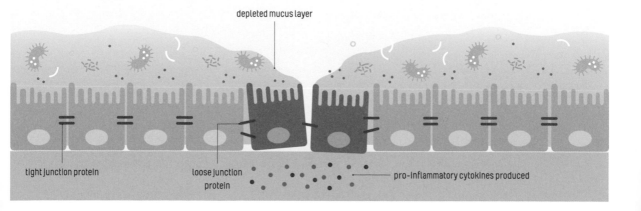

depleted mucus layer

tight junction protein

loose junction protein

pro-inflammatory cytokines produced

microbiome with the initiation and progression of many inflammatory diseases such as colorectal cancer, Crohn's disease, non-alcoholic fatty liver disease, metabolic syndrome, diabetes, obesity and atherosclerosis.

Toxins

Our environment is becoming increasingly toxic – in the air we breathe, the food we eat and what we put on our skin. Some of the biggest concerns are pesticides, pollution, heavy metals and chemicals in plastics, cosmetics and home-cleaning products.

From an evolutionary standpoint, our bodies are well equipped to deal with toxins, both from our environment and from the metabolic by-products of our bodies' own internal processes. The body has sophisticated methods of detoxing and eliminating harmful toxins. However, as our environment becomes more toxic, our bodies are struggling to keep up. Persistent, low-level exposure to toxins has a highly destructive effect on our ability to function – our body must use precious resources (such as antioxidants and vitamins) to neutralize and eliminate toxins. If our body is overwhelmed or lacks the resources to eliminate certain toxins (such as mercury leached from amalgam fillings or BPA from plastic containers), harmful toxins will start to

build up. A high toxic load can drive and perpetuate chronic inflammation.

The good news is that you can shield yourself by changing your consumer habits. This is important not only to preserve your health, but to nurture the natural ecosystems that are suffering as a result of our use of toxic chemicals.

Sources of toxic exposure

- Pollution (including industrial pollution and car exhaust)
- Pesticides and weedkillers
- Cosmetics
- Home-cleaning products
- Synthetic air fresheners and scented candles
- Dental amalgam fillings
- Mercury from certain fish, including tuna, swordfish, shark and king mackerel
- Tattoos
- Fire retardants in mattresses, carpets and furniture
- Nonstick cookware
- Chemicals in paint and plastic
- Chemicals in tap water (such as fluoride, lead and chlorine)
- Household mould
- Occupational exposure (for example, farmers exposed to pesticides or builders exposed to asbestos)

Genes

Many genes have been identified as having the potential to drive chronic inflammation that leads to disease (for example, inheriting mutations in the BRCA1 and BRCA2 genes can increase your risk for breast cancer). But having a certain gene or mutation doesn't mean that disease is inevitable.

In the twentieth century, the groundbreaking field of epigenetics showed how environmental factors can determine how our genes are expressed (turned on or off). This changed things irrevocably. We used to think that genes were our destiny, but now we understand genes are only responsible for about 10 per cent of disease. The other 90 per cent is due to internal and external factors which have collectively been dubbed the 'exposome'. The exposome is a measure of all exposures, such as diet, toxins, lifestyle factors and social behaviours, that can influence our genes and our biology. This means we have a huge influence on our genes, and whether or not they manifest disease.

Lifestyle factors

Lifestyle factors such as smoking, excess alcohol intake and lack of exercise can seriously impact your health, creating internal disruption that elevates your risk of chronic disease (*see also Lifestyle, pages 32–44*).

Cigarette smoke contains over 7,000 chemical compounds, including arsenic, cadmium, carbon monoxide and formaldehyde. Electronic cigarettes, or 'vapes', touted as a healthy alternative, contain an array of harmful chemicals such as propylene glycol, the same ingredient found in antifreeze. Exposure to these chemicals can inflame the body and accelerate your risk of chronic disease, especially cancer.

Physical inactivity also poses a major threat to our health. Extended periods of sitting have been associated with an increased risk of chronic disease, and also have a negative impact on circulation, lymphatic drainage and posture. Many people are now transitioning to standing desks, exercising more often and recognizing the benefits of regular 'movement breaks' throughout the day to counteract the negative effects of being too sedentary.

DIAGNOSING INFLAMMATION
BE YOUR OWN HEALTH DETECTIVE

If you are curious about your level of inflammation, you can find telltale signs on a routine blood test.

Blood tests are a particularly useful tool and contain a wealth of useful information to help you both identify and track inflammation. Although by no means an exhaustive list, here are some useful markers to look for. If any of these are elevated, this is a sign that you are dealing with inflammation. The longer inflammation continues, the more you are at risk of developing a chronic health condition.

hs-CRP

This marker measures the level of a C-reactive protein, which rises when inflammation is present. Raised levels are a risk factor for heart disease and stroke and can contribute to many other conditions that involve chronic inflammation.

Levels above 1mg/l indicate inflammation is present. Levels can rise after a meal so, for the most accurate reading, try to fast before having this blood test.

Erythrocyte sedimentation rate (ESR)

This measures the rate at which red blood cells settle to the bottom of a test tube. If ESR is elevated or on the upper end of the reference range, this can indicate inflammation. As with hs-CRP, it is non-specific, but can be used in combination with other tests and methods of diagnosis to identify the root cause of the problem.

The optimal range is below 5mm/hour for men and 10mm/hour for women. Anything above that can indicate inflammation, although the results are invalid in the presence of anaemia or pregnancy.

Ferritin

Ferritin is a protein that stores iron in the body. Ferritin levels are usually used to assess iron status, but can also be used to identify inflammation. When inflammation is present, ferritin levels tend to rise.

Levels above 236ng/ml in men and 122ng/ml in women suggests inflammation.

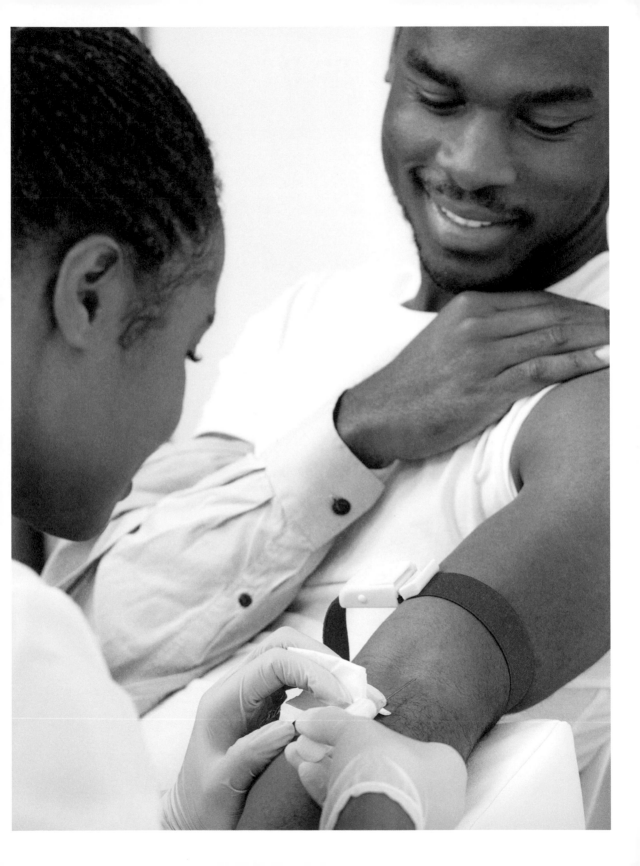

Quiz: how inflamed are you?

Working in a preventative rather than reactive manner is the most effective approach to keeping yourself well, and much of my work as a practitioner involves hunting for information and insights into a person's state of health. Information about your health will enable you to be proactive, and take action, where necessary, to stop inflammation in its tracks. The more you can understand what is going on behind the scenes, and what may be driving inflammation, the more effective you can be at keeping yourself well.

This quiz will help you get a sense of how much inflammation is present and identify key areas that are causing the most trouble.

Mark answers from 0 to 3.

0 = No, never experience this issue/symptoms don't occur
1 = Yes, occasionally
2 = Yes, occurs often
3 = Yes, all the time /symptoms are severe

Blood sugar handling

- [ ] Do you have trouble staying asleep?
- [ ] Do you feel tired, shaky, irritable or dizzy if you don't eat frequently?
- [ ] Do you feel tired after meals or have a mid-afternoon 'slump'?
- [ ] Do you crave sugar?
- [ ] Do you have a 'spare tyre' around your waist or excess abdominal fat?
- [ ] Do you need to urinate frequently?
- [ ] Do you feel thirsty all the time despite drinking water?

Total: ....

Brain and nervous system

☐ Do you feel you are forgetful or have poor short-term memory?

☐ Do you have 'brain fog' or feel 'spaced out'?

☐ Do you find it difficult to focus or concentrate?

☐ Do you experience periods of depression?

☐ Do you regularly feel anxious or startled?

☐ Do you experience severe mood swings?

☐ Do you get seasonal affective disorder (SAD) or feel low during winter?

Total: ....

Gastrointestinal system

☐ Do you experience loose bowel movements or diarrhoea?

☐ Do you experience constipation (i.e. not having a bowel movement every day, straining to have a bowel movement, have bowel movements that look like rabbit pellets or feel incomplete when you go to the toilet)?

☐ Do you notice undigested food in your stool?

☐ Do your stools float or have a light brown/tan colour?

☐ Do you get heartburn or acid reflux?

☐ Do you experience borborygmi (noisy stomach), bloating, excess wind, burping or stomach cramps?

☐ Do you have bad breath or notice a white coating on your tongue?

Total: ....

Detoxification

☐ Do you live near a busy road, airport or industrial estate?

☐ Does your job expose you to a significant number of chemicals or pollutants?

☐ Do you have acne?

☐ Do you get night sweats?

☐ Do you feel nauseous after eating, especially if you eat something rich or high in fat?

☐ Do you feel very tired, sluggish and/or get headaches the day after drinking a small amount of alcohol?

☐ Do you have a history of gallstones?

Total: ....

Adrenal and pituitary glands

☐ Do you feel dizzy if you stand up quickly?

☐ Do you get energy 'slumps' during the day, then get a second wind of energy in the evening or at nighttime?

☐ Do you feel 'wired but tired' or find it difficult to slow down and relax?

☐ Do you cry easily or find it difficult to cope with stress?

☐ Do you crave salt or salty foods such as potato crisps, chips or cheese?

☐ Do you always need sunglasses or find yourself squinting in sunlight?

☐ Is your libido low?

Total: ....

Hormones

- [ ] Do you feel cold all the time, especially in your hands and feet?

- [ ] Have you experienced excessive hair loss or hair thinning?

- [ ] Do you find it very difficult to lose weight, despite reducing calorie intake and increasing your level of exercise?

- [ ] Do you find it difficult to gain weight despite increasing your calorie intake?

- [ ] Have you noticed heart palpitations or rapid heart rate?

- [ ] Do you experience regular headaches or migraines?

- [ ] For women: do you experience painful, heavy or irregular periods?

- [ ] For men: do you experience erectile dysfunction?

Total: ....

Musculoskeletal system

- [ ] Do you frequently sit for long periods of time either at home or at work?

- [ ] Do your muscles feel weak or do you tire easily during exercise?

- [ ] Do you experience chronic neck or back pain?

- [ ] Do you notice swelling in any of your joints or muscles?

- [ ] Do you have unexplained pain and/or stiffness in various parts of your body that comes and goes?

- [ ] Do you notice clicking or popping noises coming from your joints?

- [ ] Do you feel stiff and sore after exercise and does it take a long time to recover?

Total: ....

Immune system

☐ Do you have seasonal or environmental allergies?

☐ Do you react to certain foods or have any food intolerances/sensitivities?

☐ Do you have sinus congestion or postnasal drip?

☐ Do you have a history of chronic infections such as skin infections, urinary tract infections, fungal infections, mould toxicity, glandular fever or cold sores?

☐ Do you have skin issues such as eczema, rashes or psoriasis?

☐ Do you have bronchitis or asthma?

☐ Have you had to take many antibiotics in the last ten years? (0 = none, 1 = once, 2 = three times or less, 3 = four times or more)

Total: ....

Lifestyle

☐ Do you have high stress levels?

☐ Do you smoke?

☐ Do you regularly drink alcohol?

☐ Do you regularly eat takeaway food?

☐ Do you exercise regularly? (0 = exercise daily, 1 = exercise three times a week, 2 = exercise once a week, 3 = mostly sedentary)

☐ Do you work night shifts or have a very irregular sleeping pattern?

☐ Do you get less than seven hours of sleep a night?

Total: ....

Look at your total score for each section to help identify the main areas of concern for you, and prioritize where you need to make changes.

Results

Under 2
Great news! You have little or no signs of inflammation. Now is the time to be proactive – prevention is the best medicine.

2–7
Some signs of inflammation. Read this book and decide on some simple changes you could make to target inflammation and prevent it from progressing.

8–13
Moderate level of inflammation. Your body is showing several signs of inflammation in this area. Reflect on which aspects of your lifestyle or diet might be contributing to or causing the inflammation, so you can put a strategy in place to move yourself towards better health.

14 or above
High level of inflammation. Time to take action. To avoid being overwhelmed, create an action plan by picking out two key areas in which to implement positive change over the next few weeks. Start with good food as the foundation. You may find it helpful to seek the help of a health practitioner for support.

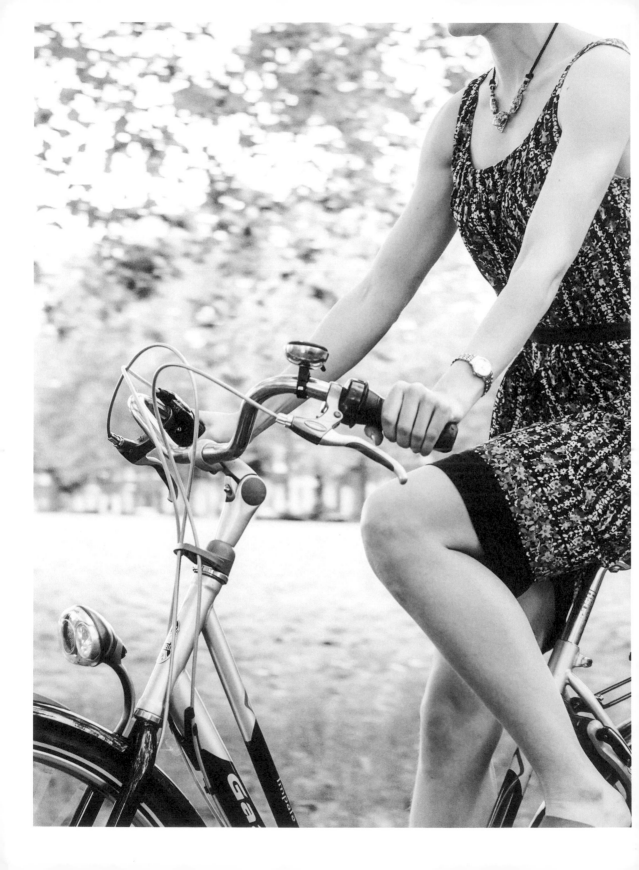

2

LIFESTYLE

In this chapter, we tackle some of the known triggers for inflammation discussed in the previous chapter, such as poor sleep, stress and exposure to toxins. We also discuss ways in which you can positively modify your lifestyle to improve your health and reduce your susceptibility to inflammation-related illnesses.

HEALTHY LIFESTYLE HABITS

Alongside diet, forming good lifestyle habits is key to reducing inflammation and preventing chronic disease.

To understand which aspects of lifestyle are the most important, consider the research conducted on 'blue zones' across the world. Blue zones are places where there are a strikingly high number of centenarians (people who live to the age of 100 and beyond) and include Okinawa in Japan, Sardinia in Italy, Nicoya in Costa Rica, Ikaria in Greece and Loma Linda in California. People in these areas not only live much longer but also have remarkably low levels of inflammation-related diseases, including obesity, cancer and heart disease. So what lifestyle factors are keeping these people so healthy and well? The shared commonalities are: natural movement throughout the day, having a purpose, relaxation or stress-relieving practices such as prayer or meditation, human connection and a sense of belonging to a community or group.

In this section, you will learn how to incorporate some of these factors into your life to create lasting, healthy habits that significantly decrease your risk for chronic inflammation and its associated diseases.

Humans are creatures of habit, and change can be hard. To kickstart the process, begin with positive changes that make you feel good. When I work with clients, I tell them to throw the 'shoulds, needs and musts' out of the window. If you're trudging to the gym once a week because you've been told you need to exercise, but you find the smell of stale sweat and blare of loud music make it a deeply unpleasant experience, it's not going to stick. Or if you're doing meditation because you think you should, but it makes you feel irritated and restless, it's clearly not the right fit. In these instances, joy is distinctly missing. Seeking healthy habits that you find enriching and will look forward to makes the process of living a healthy life so much easier and removes resistance. Joy is your most powerful tool for creating a healthy life.

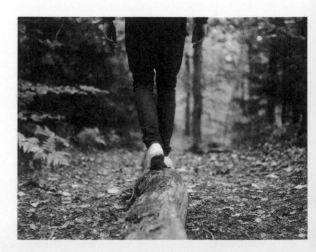

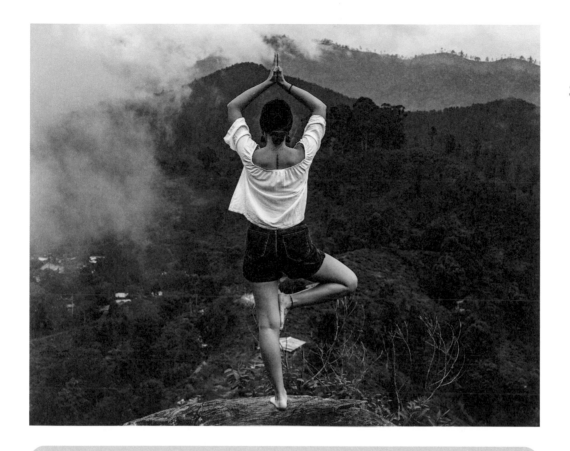

Healthy lifestyle habits

- Having a hobby/doing things you love
- Learning something new
- Breathing fresh air
- Spending time in nature
- Taking time for stillness and quiet
- Being with friends and family
- Belonging to a group or community
- Human touch, such as hugging, holding hands or getting a massage
- Regular exercise
- Quality sleep (seven to nine hours)
- Holidays/time off
- Having healthy boundaries
- Being able to say 'no' when needed
- Prioritizing your self-care and understanding that it is not self-indulgent
- Laughter
- Listening to uplifting music
- Mindfulness practices, such as meditation or breathwork
- Unplugging from social media ('tech detox')
- Decluttering your home, especially keeping your bedroom tidy and restful

STRESS

Stress can be positive or negative. Some short-term stress is useful – the excitement and sense of responsibility that come from a work promotion, for example, or the physical stress that comes from lifting weights. This is called 'eustress', which can be a vital part of helping us learn, grow and feel engaged and enthusiastic about life. Other stress, or 'distress', is destructive and results in overwhelm, anxiety and physical symptoms such as muscular tension, headaches and indigestion. Having too much stress in your life creates physiological changes in the body that can lead to chronic inflammation.

Successfully combatting stress involves finding resources that help, as well as making direct changes to the things that are causing you stress. The following tools include strategies to help you address both.

Yoga

Grounding practices such as yoga and meditation can make a huge difference in reducing stress levels. While any exercise can improve mental wellbeing, yoga is unparalleled at reducing stress and anxiety. Restorative yoga and gentle hatha yoga are particularly effective.

Meditation

A great way to start or end the day, meditation can calm your nervous system, quieten your mind and create a sense of internal spaciousness. It's a misconception that meditation involves getting rid of all thought – how difficult would that be! Meditation is in fact 'one point of focus', which means focusing on one thought, object or mantra. It is a training in presence, awareness and stillness, and is highly effective at creating a calm and balanced state of mind.

Breathwork

The breath is a powerful tool which can be used to modulate the nervous system. It is highly effective at reducing anxiety and switching our nervous system from 'fight or flight' mode to 'rest and digest' mode. Below are two of my favourite breathing techniques to use when you feel anxious or overwhelmed.

Exercise 1: Diaphragmatic breathing

1. Sit or lie down somewhere comfortable.

2. Place one hand on your belly.

3. Slowly inhale through your nose for a count of four, allowing the breath to travel right down to your abdomen. Feel your belly inflate like a balloon.

4. Slowly and with control, exhale for a count of four, allowing the belly to deflate and shrink.

5. Keep breathing for a round of ten full breaths.

Exercise 2: Box breathing

1. Inhale through your nose for a count of four. Allow the breath to travel to your abdomen rather than your chest. Keep your shoulders relaxed.

2. Hold for a count of four (avoid straining or tensing).

3. Exhale for a count of four.

4. Hold for a count of four.

5. Repeat steps 1–4 at least five times.

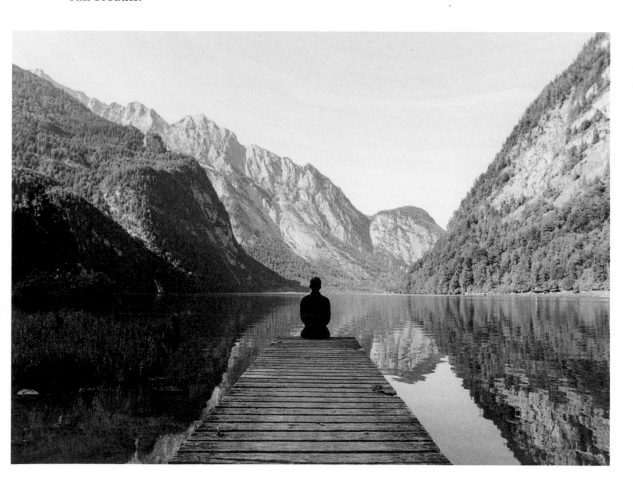

Time in nature

I've yet to meet someone who doesn't feel better after being in nature, and the results are scientifically proven. Time in nature has the power to reduce blood pressure, slow our heart rate, reduce the production of stress hormones, reduce inflammation and enhance our mental wellbeing.[1]

Scheduling 'nature dates' can be an enjoyable way to reduce your stress levels. Here are some ways to get more nature into your life:

- Take up gardening
- Adopt an exercise routine that you can do outside, such as cycling, jogging or tai chi
- Opt for time by the sea or near forests for your next holiday rather than a city break
- Try camping
- Give wild swimming a go
- Get a dog
- Have a picnic in a park
- Try forest bathing – a Japanese practice of immersing yourself in woodland and enjoying quiet contemplation of your surroundings
- Practise earthing or grounding – having direct contact with the earth, such as walking barefoot on grass
- Take your meditation practice outside – try a walking meditation in green space

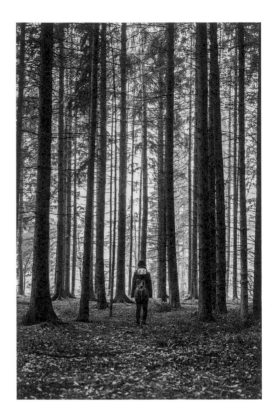

Address toxic situations, people and habits

For some people, the main source of stress comes from something toxic, such as a toxic person, a situation in their life or toxic habits that are damaging their state of mind.

Examples of toxicity include a destructive relationship, a difficult boss or self-destructive habits such as perfectionism – comparing yourself to others or putting yourself down.

James L. Wilson, the author of *Adrenal Fatigue: The 21st Century Stress Syndrome*, suggests that if you have something toxic in your life, you have three options available to you:

1. You can change the situation
2. You can change your response to the situation
3. You can leave the situation

A useful exercise is to take a fine-tooth comb to your life and consider which things are causing you stress. Make a list, as long as you like, then decide which of the three solutions above can be applied. One of the most damaging components of chronic stress is feeling overwhelmed, trapped and defeated. This exercise can put you back in the driving seat and help you make empowered decisions to move your life forward.

Detox your relationship with technology

Being glued to your phone and computer can be harmful. Scheduling downtime is the perfect antidote. This may involve taking your email off your phone, putting your phone on airplane mode after 8pm to help you unwind, or coming off all social media for a week or weekend if you feel your relationship with it has become unhealthy.

Another useful tool is to 'unfollow' all social media accounts that make you feel inadequate by comparing your work/life/weight/clothes/social life. Tidying expert Marie Kondo's approach to decluttering your household – by asking yourself if an item sparks joy and, if it doesn't, getting rid of it – can

just as effectively be applied to your social media. Ask, 'Does this spark joy?'; if not, then delete or unfollow and focus instead on the aspects of the social media that inspire or uplift you.

Self-care practices

Life requires so much from us, and the constant output of energy can leave us feeling drained and defeated. A powerful antidote to this is to seek out the services of a holistic practitioner who can help you feel nurtured and grounded.

Acupuncture, massage and craniosacral therapy are some helpful therapies, but there are many others. If you are going through a significant period of stress, having a treatment booked in once a week, or every few weeks, can give you the much-needed space to feel held and looked after. If this is unaffordable, there are many organizations that offer more economical treatments, such as low-cost multi-bed acupuncture clinics.

Life requires so much from us, and the constant output of energy can leave us feeling drained and defeated.

SLEEP

Sleep is vital, and not having enough can completely undermine your health even if your diet and exercise regime are in order. Lack of sleep can lead to increased production of the stress hormones cortisol and adrenaline, increased inflammation and insulin resistance. It can impair cognitive function, making it harder to concentrate, as well as disrupt the hormones that regulate our appetite, making weight gain more likely. We also age more quickly if we don't get enough sleep. Research has shown that lack of sleep can damage our DNA telomeres, leading to accelerated degeneration and ageing of the body. It can also increase the expression of the genes associated with chronic inflammation, heightening the risk of heart disease, cancer and diabetes.

Conversely, getting enough sleep has far-reaching benefits, including improved energy and immunity, enhanced athletic performance and decreased levels of inflammation. There's no doubt about it, sleep is powerful medicine. Prioritizing sleep is one of the best things you can do to improve your health and reduce inflammation. Let's talk about how to improve your sleep and ensure you get the most peaceful night possible.

Increasing melatonin

Melatonin is a hormone that regulates our circadian rhythm (the daily pattern that determines when it's time to sleep and when it's time to be awake). Not producing enough can impact the quality of sleep, making it harder to fall asleep or stay asleep. Certain factors can decrease your melatonin, such as:

- Exposure to blue light from computer screens or LED lighting
- Nutrient deficiencies, such as vitamin B6, folate, magnesium and zinc
- Caffeine
- Certain medications, such as beta-blockers and non-steroidal anti-inflammatory drugs (NSAIDs)

Exposure to blue light

To increase your production of melatonin, avoid blue light in the evening. Our main source in the daytime comes from sunlight, which helps regulate our circadian rhythm and keep us focused and alert. The rest of our exposure comes from phone, computer and TV screens, as well as from energy-saving light bulbs and fluorescent lighting. Blue light in the evening can trick your brain into thinking it's daytime and suppress your production of melatonin.

Eating foods that boost melatonin

To boost melatonin levels, increase your intake of foods that naturally contain melatonin, such as walnuts, cherries and olive oil. Tart cherry juice can be helpful; one 30ml (1fl oz) serving contains around 42mcg of melatonin.

Tryptophan, an essential amino acid, can be used by the body to synthesize melatonin. Tryptophan is found in protein-rich foods, such as meat, fish, chicken, eggs, nuts and beans. Eating good-quality protein at dinner can help increase your production of melatonin. Furthermore, combining tryptophan-rich foods with carbohydrate-rich foods can help tryptophan cross the blood-brain barrier (*see page 14*) more easily.

A good example of a tryptophan-boosting dinner with healthy carbohydrates is roast chicken, greens and roast squash, followed by a bowl of natural yogurt, oats, berries and chopped walnuts for dessert.

Increasing your intake of the nutrients that support melatonin production, such as vitamin B6, zinc and magnesium, can also be useful.

- **Vitamin B6-rich foods** – turkey, chicken, beef liver, salmon, cabbage, cauliflower, garlic, sweet potato
- **Zinc-rich foods** – seafood (especially oysters), beef, lamb, spinach, asparagus, almonds, cashews, sesame seeds, pumpkin seeds, shiitake mushrooms, quinoa, lentils
- **Magnesium-rich foods** – leafy greens, squash, pumpkin seeds, almonds, oats, beans, quinoa, buckwheat, brown rice

Avoid sleep disruptors

Caffeine is a stimulant and can suppress melatonin. It has a half-life of six to seven hours, so if you are struggling with sleep, it is best to avoid caffeine after lunchtime. Coffee, tea, soft drinks, energy drinks, chocolate and some cold and flu medication all contain caffeine.

Alcohol can significantly impact the quality of your sleep, causing you to wake at odd times and have increased bathroom trips due to its diuretic effect. It can also block restorative REM sleep. Avoid alcohol right before bed, and avoid it entirely if you are suffering from a period of poor sleep.

Another factor for sleep disruption is poorly managed blood sugar levels. If you're on a blood sugar rollercoaster throughout the day, this pattern can

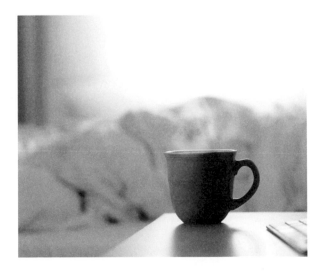

continue into the night, leading to restless sleep or waking in the middle of the night feeling hungry. Eating in a way that balances blood sugar levels throughout the day can support good sleep. If you wake up in the night feeling hungry, try a bedtime snack that stabilizes blood sugar, such as oatcakes and almond butter.

Have a bedtime wind-down routine

Having a ritual that you follow every night can be a great way to relax and prepare your body for sleep.

Try listening to a yoga nidra, a soothing form of meditation that involves a slow mental scan of different parts of the body. 'Nidra' in Sanskrit means 'sleep'. Gentle movement or stretching, such as qi gong or restorative yoga, are also excellent to do before bed. Certain herbal teas can be helpful, including chamomile and passionflower. Add two teaspoons of good-quality loose leaf chamomile or passionflower tea to a teapot and steep for two to three minutes before drinking.

I personally find an Epsom salts bath followed by a chapter of a good book to be very effective. Epsom salts contain magnesium sulphate, which helps to relax muscles and support sleep. Most people don't add enough salts to their bath to have an impact; you need 500g–1kg (1–2lb) per bath, and a 20–25-minute soak to be effective.

Sleep support checklist

- Get some sunlight exposure during the day to help regulate your circadian rhythm
- Avoid intense exercise after 8pm
- Reduce/avoid caffeine, alcohol, sugar and chocolate
- Eat melatonin-boosting foods
- Come off all screens at least one hour before bedtime
- Avoid anything stimulating before bed, such as watching the news or checking work emails
- Have a relaxing bedtime wind-down routine
- Try sleep-supporting supplements such as vitamin B6, magnesium, zinc, 5-HTP, holy basil extract, L-theanine and cannabidiol (CBD)
- Drink chamomile or passionflower tea
- Use calming essential oils such as lavender, clary sage, bergamot and Roman chamomile
- Keep your bedroom dark and cool
- Go to bed early enough to allow seven to nine hours' sleep a night

EXERCISE

The human body is not designed to be still. For thousands of years we expended a large amount of energy through physical movement throughout the day. Since the technological advances of the twentieth century, however, we have slowly become more and more sedentary.

Driving, public transport, desk jobs and computers may have made things quicker and more efficient, but they've made us significantly less healthy.

You may have heard the phrase 'sitting is the new smoking', and it is certainly true that being too sedentary increases the risk for many chronic health conditions such as heart disease, stroke, colon cancer, metabolic syndrome, type 2 diabetes and depression. Being too sedentary has a profound, negative effect on almost every area of health, from the functioning of the cardiovascular and lymphatic systems to the vitality of the immune system.

Becoming more active can positively impact chronic inflammation in a variety of ways. Regular exercise has been shown to increase the production of interleukin 6 (IL-6), a powerful anti-inflammatory protein. When you exercise, your muscle cells release IL-6, which lowers the level of several inflammatory proteins, including tumour necrosis factor (TNF) – a signalling protein produced by a variety of cells that can trigger inflammation, and interleukin-1 beta (IL 1beta), a protein produced by white blood cells which can drive up inflammation and cause damage to healthy tissue.

Exercise prevents the accumulation of inflammatory, metabolically active fat around your middle, known as visceral fat. Exercise also improves your sensitivity to insulin, which helps to reduce or prevent insulin resistance, one of the main drivers of inflammation.

It is good to aim for at least 30 minutes of exercise, five days a week. This can be any type of movement that you enjoy, including jogging, swimming, cycling, dancing, gardening, aerobics or lifting weights.

Move throughout the day

Although any amount of exercise is positive, research has shown that one session of exercise cannot offset the harm caused if you are sedentary for the rest of the day. For example, if you take a jog in the morning before work, then get in the car, spend all day at your desk, drive back from work and sit on the sofa all evening, you still have an increased risk for chronic disease. One study showed that people who sat for six hours a day had up to a 40 per cent greater risk of death from any cause compared to those who sat for three hours or fewer per day, regardless of whether they exercised or not.[2]

Here are some ideas for getting more movement into your day:

- Exercise as soon as you wake up, for example, do jumping jacks, push-ups, skipping or yoga sun salutations
- Stand – if you have a sedentary job, upgrading your desk to a standing desk is a great way to reduce the amount of time you spend sitting. You can also do calf raises or stand on a tennis ball while at your standing desk
- Keep some exercise equipment, such as resistance bands or a kettlebell, near your desk
- Have walking meetings
- Stand up or walk around for phone calls
- Stand on public transport
- Take a walk after lunch
- Get off the train or bus a stop or two earlier and walk the rest of the way
- Take the stairs instead of the lift
- Park further away from the shops and walk the rest of the way
- Stretch or use an exercise bike while watching TV

WEIGHT

Excess weight is a risk factor for many chronic health conditions, including type 2 diabetes, heart disease, arthritis, cancer and stroke.

Weight and inflammation have a two-way relationship. Excess weight can contribute to chronic inflammation, and chronic inflammation can cause weight gain and hinder weight loss. Have you ever struggled to lose weight and not understood why? The cause may be inflammation. Inflammation interferes with leptin, an important hormone that influences satiety (the feeling of being full) and helps to regulate weight. Inflammation also leads to raised cortisol levels, and cortisol significantly increases the storage of visceral fat.

Visceral fat: the worst offender

When a person gains weight, they usually increase their amount of two types of fat – subcutaneous fat and visceral fat. Subcutaneous fat is the fat just under your skin you can feel when you pinch your arms or thighs. Visceral fat is a deeper layer of fat around your abdomen that surrounds vital organs such as the pancreas, liver, stomach and intestines. Visceral fat, also known as 'angry fat', is the biggest cause for concern. This type of fat can become metabolically active and ramp up levels of inflammation by releasing hormones and inflammatory cytokines. Visceral fat can occur as a result of poor diet, stress and other factors such as alcohol, smoking and lack of exercise.

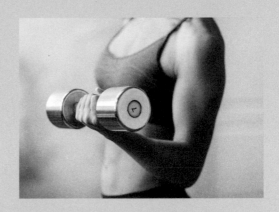

Waist to hip ratio

Measuring your waist to hip ratio is useful to identify if you have an excess of visceral fat. You can be a healthy weight but still have a high amount of visceral fat.

How to measure your waist to hip ratio:

1. Waist – use a tape measure to check the distance around your waist, starting just above the belly button.
2. Hips – measure the distance around the widest part of your hips and buttocks.
3. Divide your waist size by your hip size to calculate your waist to hip ratio.

A healthy ratio is 0.80 for women, and 0.90 for men. Anything above this indicates a high amount of visceral fat and increased risk of disease.

Optimizing weight loss

Whatever diet or weight-loss strategy you choose, ensure that you focus on meals that balance your blood sugar and insulin levels. If your blood sugar levels peak and trough too much, this can increase the likelihood of insulin resistance (*see page 18*) and hinder weight loss.

The right amount and type of exercise are important. Strength training will help you burn fat and raise your metabolic rate. Muscle tissue burns far more calories than fat tissue, and increasing your muscle mass helps to increase insulin sensitivity. It's important to avoid overtraining, however, as this can lead to insulin resistance, suppressed thyroid function and high cortisol levels – all of which can cause weight gain.

Stress can also result in weight gain. It can cause elevated cortisol levels and insulin resistance, both of which lead to increased fat storage. Incorporating a relaxation practice such as yoga or meditation can be an effective tool for lowering cortisol and accelerating weight loss.

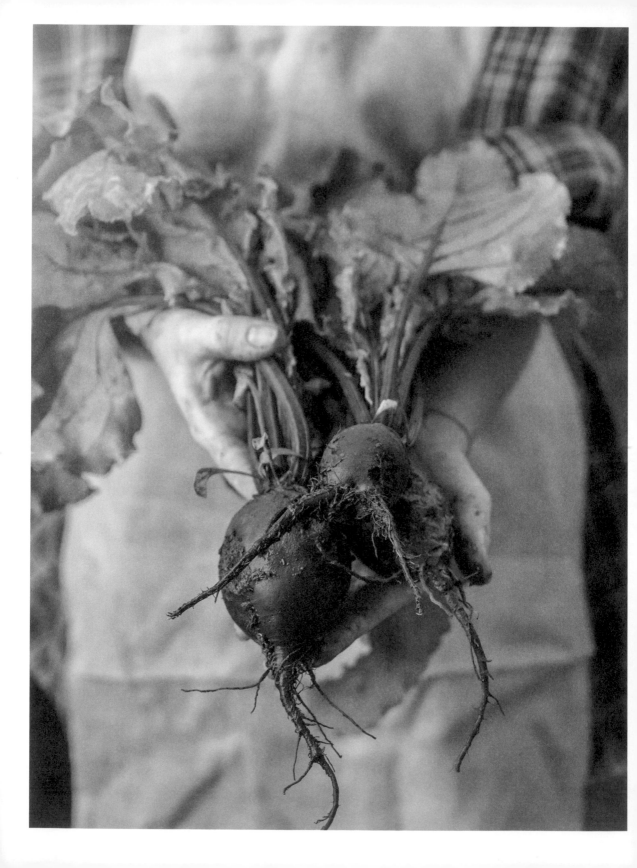

3

NUTRITION

In this chapter all aspects of food and nutrition are covered, including what to eat to support health and longevity, which cooking methods lock in nutrients and reduce the production of inflammatory compounds, and how to personalize your diet and decipher which commonly aggravating foods may be unsuitable for you. You'll discover the worst offenders for driving up inflammation and the most powerful anti-inflammatory foods to help you combat inflammation and achieve optimal health.

AN ANTI-INFLAMMATORY DIET

A healthy diet is a powerful tool to prevent inflammation and provide the raw materials needed for your body to thrive. To keep chronic inflammation at bay, the following core principles should form the foundation of your diet.

Anti-inflammatory diet principles

1. Balance your blood sugar – eat adequate protein with healthy fats, fibre and small amounts of low glycaemic load (GL) carbohydrates, such as brown rice, quinoa, buckwheat, oats, lentils, beans and sweet potato.

2. Eat a variety of fresh fruits and vegetables – aim for at least five servings of fresh vegetables a day, and one or two servings of low-sugar fruits such as berries.

3. Use herbs and spices in cooking – an easy, cheap and delicious way to upgrade the anti-inflammatory potential of your food, herbs and spices, providing an abundance of antioxidants and phytonutrients.

4. Eat plenty of healthy fats – good sources include avocados, olives, oily fish, nuts, seeds and cold-pressed oils such as olive oil and flaxseed oil.

5. Eat anti-inflammatory foods regularly – oily fish, seafood, garlic, ginger, turmeric, almonds, walnuts, chia seeds, flaxseeds, olive oil, cruciferous vegetables, tomatoes and berries.

6. Eat the best-quality food you can afford – choose organic vegetables and fruit, wild fish and seafood, pastured eggs and poultry, and grass-fed meat.

7. Use good-quality salt – rock or sea salt contains important minerals.

8. Drink plenty of water. Aim for 2 litres (3½ pints) of filtered water daily.

9. Eat prebiotic- and probiotic-rich foods that support the beneficial bacteria in your gut (*see page 51*).

10. Identify food intolerances – use an elimination diet to identify ingredients that are causing inflammation (*see pages 57–8*).

Choosing quality food

If you're feeling confused about food and health, it can be helpful to ask yourself, 'How close to nature is my food?'. Instead of getting bogged down with conflicting nutritional information, focus primarily on the *quality* of what you're eating, especially if you're just embarking on your health journey and are feeling overwhelmed. If you eat food made with fresh ingredients that have been tampered with as little as possible, you've already won half the battle.

Wild fish versus farmed fish

Wild fish have higher levels of omega-3 and lower levels of omega-6 than farmed fish. Farmed fish are higher in omega-6 as the fish are fattened on feed containing soya and corn. Wild fish are raised without the use of antibiotics, pesticides and polychlorinated biphenyls (PCBs). PCBs are chemicals added to the processed feed given to farmed fish, which disrupt our reproductive systems and increase the risk of cancer.

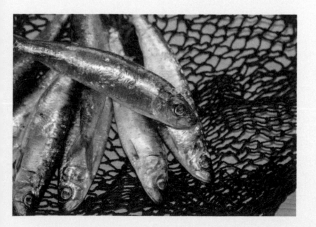

Avoiding mercury in fish

Some fish contain dangerous levels of mercury. Generally the larger and older the fish, the more mercury is stored in its tissues, as mercury bioaccumulates over time. Avoid the following fish:

- Bluefish
- Grouper
- King mackerel
- Marlin
- Orange roughy
- Shark
- Swordfish
- Tilefish from the Gulf of Mexico
- Tuna

Choosing meat

Meat provides a concentrated source of nutrition, including protein, vitamin B12 and iron. But not all meat is created equal.

Factory-farmed meat is completely different from grass-fed or pastured meat. Factory-farmed animals are raised in shockingly poor conditions and fattened on a diet of refined grains, a far cry from their natural diet. Bad diets make for sick animals, and sick humans too. Factory-farmed animals are also given antibiotics and growth hormones which end up in our food, playing havoc with our gut flora and increasing our risk for cancer.

Make good-quality meat a priority, not only for health, but for environmental and ethical reasons too.

Making quality food more affordable

Here are some ways to make good-quality food more affordable:

- Use the Environment Working Group's Clean Fifteen™ and Dirty Dozen™ lists (*see www.ewg.org/foodnews/4*). Updated annually, they rank the pesticide contamination in fruits and vegetables. Prioritize buying organic versions of the most contaminated foods on the list

- Organic veg box schemes provide you with weekly vegetables direct from a farmer. The produce is seasonal, local and tends to be cheaper than buying from the supermarket

- Growing your own produce is very gratifying and a lovely way to connect with food more deeply. If you don't have a garden space, there are some great indoor growing kits for items like herbs, tomatoes and chillies

- Choose cheaper varieties of oily fish, such as sardines, anchovies and mackerel, rather than fish like salmon

- Eat cheaper cuts of meat. Better-quality meat (organic and pastured or grass fed) is undoubtedly expensive, but you can buy cheaper cuts of meat, such as beef brisket rather than steaks or chicken thighs rather than breasts

- Batch-cook large portions and freeze to save money and reduce waste

Nutrient-rich foods

Healthy fats

Healthy fat is essential for good health and a key player in preventing chronic inflammation. Fats are needed for our cell membranes, to protect us from harmful toxins, balance blood sugar, maintain the health of the brain, eyes and skin and to regulate our hormones. Fats also aid the absorption of fat-soluble vitamins A, D, E and K, which are crucial for a healthy immune system.

Omega-6 and omega-3

Omega-6 and omega-3 fatty acids are known as 'essential fatty acids' because our body can't produce them. We need omega-6 for the initiation of the inflammatory response (we don't want to get rid of inflammation completely – *see pages 10–11*), and also for the resolution of inflammation. We also need omega-3 both to reduce and resolve inflammation.

Our ancestors had a ratio of omega-6 to omega-3 close to 1:1 or 2:1. However, since the introduction of vegetable oils into our diet, the ratio has been very different – closer to 15:1, and in some cases as high as 50:1.[1] Refined vegetable oils and the processed foods that contain them have contributed to this unbalanced ratio and the prevalence of chronic inflammatory conditions. They not only skew the omega-6 to omega-3 ratio, which drives inflammation, but increase inflammation by creating oxidative stress (*see page 17*).

Research suggests that the ideal ratio is 4:1 or below. We can achieve this by eating healthy sources of omega-6 (found in nuts, seeds, eggs and olive oil) and plenty of omega-3 (in fish and seafood). If you're vegan, you can eat plant foods such as flaxseeds, hemp, chia seeds and walnuts, which contain good amounts of omega-3, but in the alpha-lipoic acid (ALA) form. ALA can be converted into eicosapentaenoic acid (EPA) or docosahexaenoic acid (DHA), but the conversion process isn't always efficient in humans. ALA, EPA and DHA are all omega-3 fatty acids, but DHA and EPA are the biologically active forms of omega-3, and therefore more important for fighting inflammation. Another alternative for vegans is to take an omega-3 supplement made from algae oil, which naturally contains EPA and DHA.

To avoid excessively high omega-6 levels, avoid all refined vegetable oils (*see page 17*). This will ensure that the ratio stays within a healthy range.

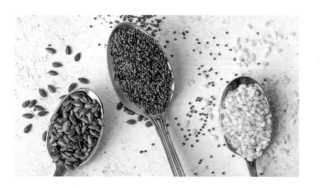

Good gut health

Modern diets and the widespread use of antibiotics have lead to imbalances in our gut bacteria and a general decline in their diversity. Fortunately, there's lots we can do to support our gut microbiota, particularly prebiotic- and probiotic-rich foods, and resistant starch.

Prebiotics provide a food source for our gut bacteria and probiotics provide an abundance of live micro-organisms that can benefit our health. Resistant starch is a type of starch that travels through the gut undigested until it reaches our large intestine, where our gut bacteria use it as a food source to produce short-chain fatty acids, which fuel and maintain the cells lining our colon. Eat more of the following foods to support your gut microbiota:

- Prebiotic-rich foods – garlic, onions, leeks, broccoli, artichokes, asparagus, beetroot, chicory root, oats, rice, legumes, almonds, apples, berries, cacao, green tea, olive oil

- Probiotic-rich (fermented) foods – kefir, live yogurt, kimchi, kvass, sauerkraut, beetroot, apple cider vinegar, miso

- Resistant starch – oats, rice, potatoes, green bananas, plantain, legumes (Cooling rice, potatoes and legumes after cooking significantly increases the amount of resistant starch)

Healthy cooking methods

To keep inflammation at bay, minimize high-heat cooking methods such as barbecuing, frying, grilling and roasting – especially where the food becomes browned or charred. High-heat cooking can lead to the formation of harmful compounds such as advanced glycation end-products (AGEs) and heterocyclic amines (HCAs), which can cause oxidative stress, increase the risk of cancer and accelerate ageing.

The healthiest cooking methods are poaching, steaming and boiling. Boiling does result in a greater loss of nutrients than steaming, as nutrients leach into the water. Sautéing and stir-frying in a healthy oil retain nutrients but result in less harmful compounds than barbecuing, grilling, and so on.

Oils to use in cooking

Some oils are better than others for cooking because of the difference in their smoke points. Heating an oil past its smoke point can destroy precious phytochemicals and lead to the production of inflammatory compounds. Depending on the cooking process, use the following oils:

- For higher-heat cooking – avocado oil, macadamia nut oil, ghee

- For low–medium heat cooking – extra virgin olive oil , butter

- For adding to foods when serving – extra virgin olive oil, flaxseed oil, walnut oil, avocado oil, pumpkin seed oil, macadamia nut oil

Anti-inflammatory swaps for common foods

Avoid these:	Replace with these:
Refined fats and oils: vegetable oil, rapeseed oil, corn oil, grapeseed oil, sunflower oil, safflower oil, peanut oil, margarine	Olive oil, avocado oil, coconut oil, walnut oil, flaxseed oil (all should be extra virgin or cold pressed); grass-fed butter and ghee; tallow/lard
Dairy	Unsweetened almond milk, coconut milk, hemp milk, hazelnut milk, macadamia milk, Brazil nut milk, oat milk; coconut, almond or cashew yogurt; coconut water; kefir; nut cheese; oat cream; coconut cream

Gluten	Buckwheat, quinoa, amaranth or brown rice bread. If gluten is tolerated, sprouted wheat or rye bread
Conventional meat and poultry and processed meat and poultry	Organic grass-fed or grass-finished meat; organic pastured chicken
Farmed fish and seafood	Wild-caught fish and seafood
Non-organic, unfermented soya products	Organic, fermented soya: miso, natto, tempeh, tamari
Refined sugar and artificial sweeteners: acesulfame, aspartame, neotame, saccharin and sucralose	Stevia, fresh or dried fruits; cinnamon, wild honey, maple syrup, coconut sugar, blackstrap molasses as an occasional treat
Table salt	Natural rock or sea salt
Soft drinks including diet versions	Kombucha, sparkling water with a slice of lemon, coconut water
Potato crisps	Kale chips, oat cakes, buckwheat crackers, seaweed crisps, nuts, vegetable crudités
Chips	Potato salad or boiled new potatoes (even better if eaten the next day to allow resistant starch to develop)
Mashed potato	Cauliflower mash
Pasta	Courgetti or brown rice pasta
Cereal	Overnight bircher muesli, chia seed porridge, porridge
Peanut butter	Almond butter, walnut butter, hazelnut butter, pecan butter, tahini, pumpkin seed butter (raw/unroasted)
Protein powders with sugar or artificial sweeteners	Pure whey, pea, hemp or brown rice protein (unsweetened or sweetened with stevia)
Tap water	Filtered water, mineral or spring water from glass bottles

POTENTIALLY INFLAMMATORY FOODS

Some foods have the potential to cause inflammation, depending on the quality and whether you tolerate them. To help navigate this, let's look at three food groups that create the most confusion.

Dairy

From a nutritional perspective, dairy is a rich source of vitamins and minerals, especially vitamin D and calcium. But more and more people report feeling worse when they consume dairy. Why is this happening when our ancestors comfortably consumed dairy for thousands of years?

Firstly, the quality of the dairy we now consume is poor. Conventional dairy (non grass-fed, non organic) contains pesticides, steroids, growth hormones and antibiotics due to the way the animals are reared. The pasteurization process destroys the naturally occurring lactase enzyme that helps break down lactose. Raw, organic, grass-fed dairy is completely different. It has many health-giving properties, and is often far better tolerated. The difficulty with raw dairy is that it is not easy to find, and there are safety concerns around bacterial contamination.

Secondly, for many people, whether or not they tolerate dairy boils down to the health of their gut. Gut issues such as intestinal permeability (leaky gut syndrome) or small intestinal bacterial overgrowth (a common cause of IBS) increase the likelihood of reacting react to dairy. Additionally, sensitivity to gluten increases the chances of reacting to dairy due to cross-reactivity, where the immune system mistakes milk proteins for gluten and mounts an inflammatory response. Considering the high number of people struggling with compromised gut function, it's not surprising that many feel better when they remove dairy from their diet.

If this all sounds confusing, the best solution is to investigate for yourself whether dairy suits you by trying an elimination diet (*see pages 57–8*). If you reintroduce dairy and don't notice any symptoms, then good-quality dairy may be a healthful part of your diet. Good choices include organic grass-fed butter or ghee, which contain minimal lactose but a high amount of butyrate, a short-chain fatty acid with many anti-inflammatory benefits. Organic natural yogurt and kefir also contain beneficial bacteria that can support your gut health, and whey protein provides powerful immunoglobulins that can strengthen the immune system.

Gluten

For many years it was argued that the only people who needed to avoid gluten were those with coeliac disease. Luckily, the tide has turned and non-coeliac gluten sensitivity is now a medically recognized condition. For those affected, it can drive low-grade chronic inflammation and create many unpleasant symptoms, including joint pain, chronic fatigue, brain fog, digestive issues and anaemia.[2]

Research has demonstrated that gluten (especially a protein component of gluten called gliadin) can cause intestinal permeability. A compromised gut lining can lead to improperly digested food particles leaking into the bloodstream and provoking an immune response (*see page 21*). The inflammation caused can lead to a multitude of non-specific symptoms throughout the body and, over time, can completely degrade a person's health and vitality.

Wheat and other gluten-containing grains have been cultivated for human consumption for some 10,000 years, so

why are more and more people becoming intolerant? There are a few theories. Some argue that modern strains of wheat have been modified and contain new allergenic components that weren't present in ancient wheat strains. Others point towards our increasingly disrupted gut flora as a potential cause, or the fact that most grains are heavily sprayed with harmful pesticides. Additionally, we have moved away from traditional methods of preparing grains, including sprouting and fermenting, which can make them more digestible.

Regardless of the cause, many people feel significantly better on a gluten-free diet. Some notice skin rashes or sinus congestion melt away; others notice a dramatic shift in their health – depression, brain fog, stubborn abdominal fat – all gone. It is worth trying a gluten-free elimination diet (*see pages 57–8*) for three weeks to see how you feel.

The pitfalls of a gluten-free diet

The number of people trying a gluten-free diet has exploded in recent years, and many companies have cashed in on the trend by churning out 'free-from' products. But gluten free doesn't necessarily equal healthy. Most gluten-free products that you find in the supermarket are highly processed, devoid of nutrients and bear no resemblance to a natural food. If you try a gluten-free diet, it's essential that you source brands that don't rely on a lengthy list of artificial ingredients, preservatives and added sugars (often called something misleading such as rice syrup or treacle). I suggest getting to know your local health food shop – they often sell better-quality gluten-free products than supermarkets. Making your own gluten-free bread is also a good option; it's cheaper and you know exactly what's going in it.

Soya

Soya is another food that brings confusion. Whether soya is good or bad comes mostly down to the quality. Processed soya is extremely unhealthy and should be avoided as much as possible. Processed soya products include soya protein isolate, soya cheese, soya ice cream, soya meat substitutes and soya bean oil.

Countries that traditionally eat soya tend to consume wholefood, fermented forms of soya such as miso, tempeh and natto. These foods are a great source of vitamin K (which you don't get in unfermented soya), minerals and protein, and the fermentation process improves digestibility and reduces anti-nutrients such as phytic acid (which can interfere with the absorption of minerals).

If you suspect you may be reacting to soya, try the elimination diet (*see pages 57–8*) to confirm whether you should keep it in your diet.

Foods to avoid

The following foods are the worst offenders for fanning the flames of inflammation:

- Sugar
- Artificial sweeteners – acesulfame, aspartame, neotame, saccharin and sucralose
- Refined carbohydrates – white flour, chips, potato crisps, biscuits, cakes, desserts, breakfast cereals, pizza
- Refined fats and oils and trans fats (found in vegetable oils and margarine)
- Factory-farmed meat
- High-mercury fish such as tuna and swordfish
- Genetically modified soya, processed soya products (including meat substitutes and anything containing soya protein isolate)
- Processed 'free-from' products that are high in sugar and artificial ingredients
- Food additives (such as sodium benzoate, sodium nitrate, BHA and BHT, MSG and carrageenan)
- Artificial food colourings

WHAT ELSE CAN HELP?

There is no universally perfect diet that will suit everyone– no 'one size fits all'.

Blood type, genetics, metabolic rate, climate, underlying state of health (especially gut health) and lifestyle all interweave to form a complex web of factors that determine the diet that will best support your health. The foods that you thrive on may make another person feel lethargic, bloated and gain weight. This is why it is important to experiment with different styles of eating to help you crack the code of which foods make you feel best. The first step is to identify the foods that make you feel bad and give you symptoms. One of the best methods for this is an elimination diet.

The elimination diet

Identifying foods that are aggravating your body is a key step in getting rid of chronic inflammation. Many food intolerance tests are poor quality and unreliable, and the ones that are more advanced can be prohibitively expensive. The elimination diet is a good alternative to help you find out which foods may be disrupting your health.

The purpose of an elimination diet:

- **Identifies food triggers** – helps you to clearly identify food triggers that are aggravating your immune system, so you can create a more tailored diet.

- **Reduces inflammation** – food reactions can trigger inflammation in the gut and make the gut lining more permeable. Intestinal permeability can lead to further inflammation as bacteria and toxins are able to leak from the intestine into the blood-stream and trigger the immune system. By removing offending foods you can reduce inflammation and give the gut lining a chance for repair.

- **Encourages a greater level of awareness to food** – an elimination diet encourages you to tune in and listen to your body. The body can't speak but it does still communicate through symptoms. Going through the elimination process will help you to focus on listening and observing to see how your body responds to certain foods. This leads to a greater understanding and connection with your body and a motivation to want to work in partnership.

You may already suspect specific foods and want to investigate with an elimination diet, or perhaps you have strange, unexplained symptoms and want to see if there is any link with food. You can either choose a handful of foods from the common food triggers list below to trial, or remove all the foods if you think you may be reacting to several different foods. For many, gluten and dairy are the main culprits and they feel markedly better after the elimination diet.

Common food triggers:

- Gluten-containing grains (wheat, rye, barley, and oats unless specified as gluten-free oats)
- Dairy
- Eggs
- Corn
- Soya
- Peanuts

How to do an elimination diet

1. Choose which foods to eliminate (they don't need to be the foods listed above), then plan your diet. Prepare well and sketch out a rough menu plan to ensure you have a variety of healthy options for meals and snacks.

2. Remove suspected foods for three weeks. Complete avoidance is important to calm any inflammation and get clear results when you reintroduce the foods. Observe your body and track your symptoms throughout the process.

3. After three weeks, choose one food (say, dairy) to reintroduce and eat two to three generous portions of that food each day for two days. During these two days, observe to see if you have any symptoms such as fatigue, joint pain, headaches, skin complaints, increased heart rate, stomach pain, bowel movement changes, bloating or irritability. If there are symptoms when you reintroduce the food, this is a sign that it isn't suiting you and you should continue to avoid it. If there are no symptoms and you feel fine, this food should be okay to eat.

4. On the third day, you can move onto reintroducing the next food, as long as any symptoms caused by introducing the first food have calmed down.

Do I have to avoid the foods that I react to forever?

Not necessarily. Some people find that after eliminating offending foods for a period of time, and working to address underlying issues such as intestinal permeability and microbial imbalances, they can safely bring back certain foods into their diet.

A blood sugar balanced diet

Insulin resistance is a major cause of chronic inflammation (*see pages 18–19*). Many people have wildly fluctuating blood sugar levels and the early signs of insulin resistance without even realizing it. How do you know if this applies to you? Here are some signs that your blood sugar is poorly managed:

- Fatigue (especially energy dips such as an afternoon 'slump')
- Feeling irritable/dizzy/shaky if you don't eat every couple of hours
- Sugar cravings
- Needing caffeine to get through the day
- Restless sleep
- Frequent urination
- Excessive thirst
- Difficulty losing weight
- Fat storage around the midriff
- Brain fog

How your blood sugar levels fluctuate throughout the day is called glycaemic variability. Poor glycaemic variability is characterized by a rollercoaster of blood sugar levels, which can lead to unpleasant symptoms and increased susceptibility for insulin resistance, metabolic syndrome and diabetes. Balancing blood sugar levels is not only crucial for reducing inflammation, it also makes you feel good – giving you consistent energy, sharp focus and restful sleep.

Causes of imbalanced blood sugar levels:

- Eating too much sugar and simple or refined carbohydrates
- Eating too many carbohydrates without enough protein, fat and fibre to balance
- Chronic stress
- Too much or too little exercise

Get off the rollercoaster

To balance blood sugar levels, swap refined carbohydrates (such as biscuits, white bread, cereal, cakes, potato chips) for small amounts of complex carbohydrates such as brown rice, squash, sweet potato, quinoa and oats.

Another important cornerstone for balancing blood sugar is eating enough protein with meals. Although individual requirements vary, a useful visual guide is to ensure that your protein serving is roughly the size of your palm. Good sources of protein include meat, fish, poultry, eggs, ancient grains such as quinoa and millet, pulses and beans.

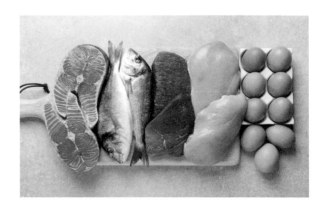

Fat and fibre are also key, as they stabilize blood sugar levels by slowing down the digestion and absorption of carbohydrates. Healthy sources of fat include olive oil, olives, avocado, nuts, seeds and oily fish. Fibre is found in abundance in all vegetables, with non-starchy vegetables being the best choice for blood sugar stabilization.

To give you a sense of what it looks like to be on or off the blood sugar rollercoaster, here are some examples:

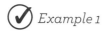 *Example 1*

Breakfast – boiled egg and avocado on buckwheat bread
Lunch – quinoa salad with walnuts
Dinner – baked trout, butternut squash, steamed broccoli and olive oil
Snack – blueberries with coconut yogurt, cinnamon and chopped Brazil nuts

 Example 2

Breakfast – coffee, granola with banana, honey and low-fat milk
Lunch – sandwich and potato crisps, mango smoothie
Dinner – pasta with tomato sauce and cheese
Snack – coffee, chocolate rice cakes

Harness the power of natural foods

Adding herbs and spices, in particular fenugreek, cinnamon and turmeric, to food can help to reduce blood sugar levels and improve insulin sensitivity.

Apple cider vinegar is also effective at preventing blood sugar spikes after meals and improving insulin sensitivity. One study demonstrated that 20ml (about four teaspoons) of apple cider vinegar before a carbohydrate-rich meal improved insulin sensitivity by 34 per cent.[3]

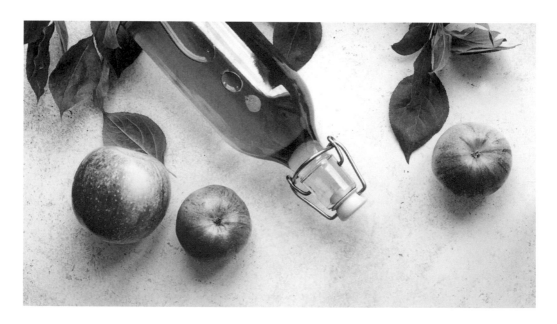

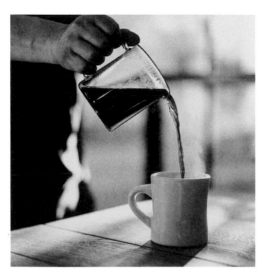

Ditch the caffeine

Too much caffeine can lead to unbalanced blood sugar levels. Your morning coffee may not be working for you if you find yourself full of beans one minute and shaky, hungry and irritable the next. If you have noticed any of the symptoms mentioned, try two weeks without caffeine and compare how you feel.

A vegan diet

The vegan diet has exploded in popularity in recent years. But is it the best choice for fighting inflammation? Not necessarily.

A vegan diet that is filled with sugar, processed meat substitutes and refined carbohydrates will hike up inflammation just as much as an unhealthy diet that contains animal foods. In fact, it is more likely to cause inflammation if nutritionally dense foods such as meat and eggs are replaced with refined grains and vegetable oils – the mainstays of convenience vegan foods.

It's also difficult to get everything you need on a vegan diet without careful planning. Many vegan diets are lacking in protein, zinc, iron, calcium, iodine, vitamins D and B12.

It's impossible to get enough B12 on a vegan diet without eating fortified foods or taking a supplement. As for the anti-inflammatory omega-3 fats, there are ALA-rich foods such as chia, hemp, edamame and walnuts, but the conversion from ALA to omega-3 is not always efficient (*see page 51*).

If you choose to go vegan for ethical or environmental reasons, or just because you want to see how you feel, then focus on eating an abundance of anti-inflammatory vegetables, fruits and herbs and plenty of protein with every meal; also increase your intake of plant-based sources of zinc, iron, calcium and iodine, and consider supplementing with vitamins D, B12 and plant-based omega-3 from algae.

In this section we look at individual foods that have powerful anti-inflammatory properties. Although all fresh whole foods can promote good health, research has shown that the following foods in particular are a cut above the rest for fighting inflammation.

Turmeric

Turmeric comes from *Curcuma longa,* a flowering plant that belongs to the ginger family. Native to India and Southeast Asia, its medicinal properties have been celebrated for centuries. The turmeric spice itself is found underground, in the rhizome, or root-like stem of the plant. There are over 50 names for turmeric in the ancient Indian language of Sanskrit, including *jayanti*, meaning 'one that wins over diseases', and *bhadra*, meaning 'lucky'.[4]

One of the most powerful ingredients in your anti-inflammatory armoury, turmeric has many scientifically proven benefits and can even rival some anti-inflammatory drugs, without the unpleasant side effects.[5][6][7] The reason turmeric is so useful for inflammation is largely due to the chemical compound curcumin, which gives turmeric its distinctive colour.

Health benefits of curcumin

Due to its potent anti-inflammatory effect, curcumin has been shown to be useful for many different conditions, including arthritis, depression, hayfever and non-alcoholic fatty liver disease. It can directly target inflammation by blocking pro-inflammatory signalling molecules such as nuclear factor kappa B (NF-Kb) and interleukin 8 (IL-8).[8]

As a powerful antioxidant, curcumin can help to mop up oxidative stress in the body, as well as boost the activity of your body's own antioxidant enzymes such as glutathione and superoxide dismutase (SOD).[9]

Curcumin can also boost levels of brain-derived neurotrophic factor (BDNF), a protein that preserves and stimulates the growth of brain cells, therefore improving and protecting brain function.[10]

How to improve bioavailability

When consuming turmeric, it is difficult for the body to absorb and utilize all of the available curcumin. Fortunately, the absorption can be improved by adding fat and black pepper. Curcumin is fat soluble, so consuming it alongside fat means the curcumin is more likely to be absorbed into your bloodstream. Black pepper is helpful due to its high content of piperine, a phytochemical that improves the absorption of curcumin and slows the rate at which it is broken down in the liver (therefore increasing the amount of curcumin present in the bloodstream).

TIP: When consuming turmeric, combine it with black pepper and some healthy fat such as coconut oil, ghee or avocado. The fat and black pepper combination can increase the bioavailability of curcumin by up to 2,000 per cent!

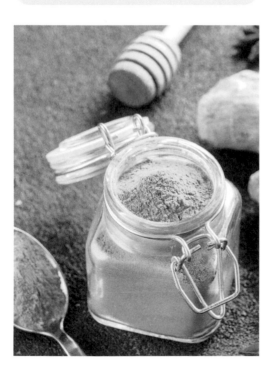

How to use turmeric

Turmeric can be used fresh or dried (careful with fresh turmeric – it will give you *very* orange hands!). It's a versatile ingredient with a mild, pleasant taste, and can therefore be incorporated into a wide variety of different dishes. Here are some ideas to help you increase your intake of turmeric:

- Juice fresh turmeric and drink on its own or add other anti-inflammatory ingredients such as lemon and ginger

- Make a 'golden milk' drink (*see page 86*)

- Include in a salad dressing

- Add to soups

- Add to smoothies

- Mix into energy balls with dates, nuts and coconut oil

- Use it for baking muffins. Banana and turmeric go nicely together

- Blend into butter with ground cinnamon and ginger to make a delicious spread

- Sprinkle on scrambled eggs or add to an omelette

- Dust on vegetables before roasting

- Use turmeric in curries. It partners really well with coconut milk

- Make turmeric tea by mixing 1 teaspoon of dried turmeric with the juice of 1 lemon, honey and hot water

Ginger

A superstar of the plant world, ginger can be distinguished by its strong, fiery taste (drink some raw ginger juice and you'll see what I mean!). Ginger has long been recognized for its medicinal and therapeutic properties. It originated in Southeast Asia over 5,000 years ago, and is now appreciated worldwide as a culinary spice and therapeutic agent. Fresh ginger root contains over 100 bioactive compounds, but the majority of its health benefits come from a chemical compound called gingerol.

Health benefits of ginger

Ginger is an excellent digestive aid because to its ability to reduce gas and relax the intestinal tract. It is a useful remedy for alleviating nausea and vomiting – its effectiveness at relieving motion sickness, chemotherapy-induced nausea and morning sickness has been well documented. [11][12]

Ginger can also support cardiovascular health, boost testosterone levels in men, improve memory and protect the liver. It can

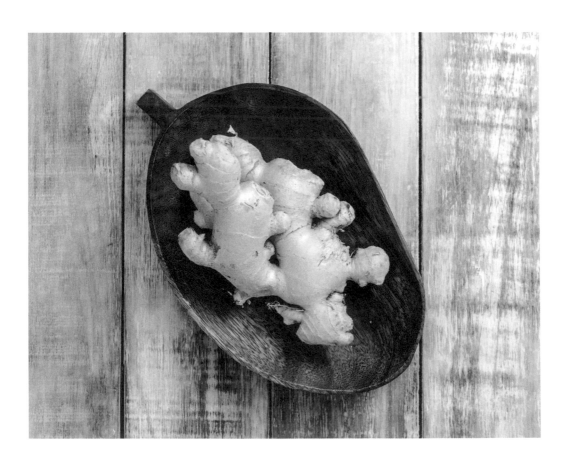

block the pro-inflammatory NF-kB pathway the signalling molecules that tell the body to launch an inflammatory response), reduce the activity of inflammatory genes and reduce the production of pain and inflammation-causing chemicals. For this reason, ginger can be helpful in managing many inflammatory conditions, including arthritis, migraines and menstrual pain. Research has demonstrated that, at certain doses, ginger can match the effectiveness of non-steroidal anti-inflammatory drugs (NSAIDs) such as aspirin and ibuprofen. This is promising, particularly as drugs used to treat pain and inflammation can damage the stomach and intestinal lining if used very frequently or long term.

Ginger contains a huge amount of antioxidants, more than any vegetables or fruit, surpassed only by pomegranates and some types of berries.[13] It can also protect our bodies' own antioxidants, including two of our most powerful – glutathione and superoxide dismutase (SOD).[14] Too much oxidative stress (free radicals) in the body can trigger inflammation. The antioxidants in ginger help to counteract this, acting as a powerful tool against excess inflammation.

How to use ginger

- Add fresh or ground ginger to smoothies and soups

- Juice fresh ginger alongside other anti-inflammatory ingredients

- Juice fresh ginger and make into an immune-supportive tea with hot water, lemon and honey

- Combine with other aromatic spices in tagines

- Add ground ginger and cinnamon to fruit compotes

- Use fresh ginger in stir-fries, ramen and curries

- Mix finely grated fresh ginger and miso paste to coat vegetables before grilling

- Use in baking – ginger and carrot complement each other nicely

- Infuse fresh ginger into an oil and apply topically to help soothe aching muscles or arthritis

Green tea

One of the healthiest drinks on the planet, green tea is a rich source of antioxidants, vitamins and minerals, and an excellent choice to include in your anti-inflammatory food pharmacy.

Health benefits of green tea

Green tea is a rich source of polyphenols. Polyphenols are plant chemicals that have powerful anti-inflammatory properties and a host of health benefits. One of the most beneficial polyphenols in green tea is called epigallocatechin gallate (EGCG). Polyphenols have an antioxidant effect, helping to mop up free radicals and reduce oxidative stress. By reducing free-radical production, they prevent inflammation and protect against a number of diseases. Polyphenols can also increase the growth of beneficial bacteria in the gut microbiota, which can guard against chronic inflammation.

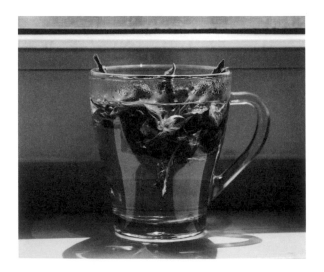

TIP: Avoid pouring boiling water directly onto the green tea as it can alter the taste and damage the precious phytochemicals. Leave your water to sit for ten minutes after boiling then pour over the tea. Leave it to brew for one minute before drinking.

Green tea can enhance cognitive function due to the presence of EGCG, caffeine, and L-theanine. The levels of caffeine are much lower than in coffee, and any stimulating effect is mitigated by L-theanine, a calming amino acid that, aside from improving focus, helps to promote relaxation and improves sleep. Hence most people who drink green tea report more stable energy levels and increased mental clarity throughout the day compared to when they drink coffee.

Research suggests that green tea can play a role in reducing the risk of several types of cancers, prevent diabetes, improve dental health and increase longevity. Green tea can also help to reduce your LDL cholesterol levels (the 'bad' cholesterol). Studies indicate that it can reduce your risk of cardiovascular disease by up to 31 per cent.[15]

Green tea is also useful if you're trying to lose weight as it can increase your metabolic rate and promote fat burning.[16]

Choosing green tea

When choosing green tea look for a high-quality, organic loose leaf green tea. There are many different types of green tea to choose from, but Japanese Sencha green tea is a good one to look out for as it tends to contain the lowest level of pollutants and the highest levels of antioxidants.

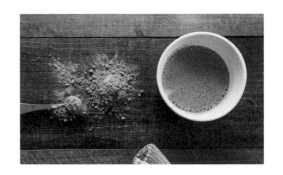

How to use green tea

- Infuse green tea in hot water and enjoy it as it is

- Cold brew green tea in cold water for 12–15 hours

- Make a refreshing lemonade with green tea, lemon juice, ice, water and a natural sweetener such as stevia

- In winter, make a matcha latte and a frappé in summer

- Mix matcha into fresh vegetable juices

- Add matcha to smoothies

- Add matcha to homemade chocolate

- Use matcha in baking

- Mix matcha into pancake batter

- Make matcha energy balls along with dates, nuts and desiccated coconut

- Try a panna cotta with matcha, vanilla extract or paste and coconut milk

- Cook ochazuke, a rice dish that is steeped in green tea

Green tea and matcha: what is the difference?

Green tea leaves and matcha powder both come from the same plant, *Camellia sinensis*. They can have different nutritional profiles due to processing methods. Matcha powder is made from green tea leaves that have been ground into a fine powder. Matcha is grown in the shade, forcing the plant to produce more chlorophyll to better convert any sunlight that reaches the plant into energy, whereas most green tea plants are grown in the sun. Shade-growing results in more nutrients, more antioxidants and a stronger flavour. Additionally, matcha powder dissolves in water, so you consume the entire leaves (and all their nutrition) rather than just infused water. Both have excellent anti-inflammatory qualities, but matcha is more concentrated and tends to be more expensive.

Oily fish

All types of fish contain nutrients that are beneficial for health, but they are more potent in oily fish. Oily fish contain a large amount of oil in their tissues and belly cavity, whereas white fish (non-oily fish), such as cod or sea bass, only contain oil in the liver, and the total levels of oil are much lower.

Health benefits of oily fish

Oily fish is a rich source of omega-3 fatty acids (*see page 50*). It contains two types of omega-3, EPA and DHA, which have potent anti-inflammatory effects. Oily fish is also a great source of protein, as well as immune-supporting nutrients vitamins A and D, zinc and selenium.

Omega-3 fats have been shown to be useful in many different areas of health and are a very effective tool for lowering inflammation. Increasing intake of EPA and DHA can be helpful for a number of autoimmune and chronic inflammatory diseases such as rheumatoid arthritis, lupus, inflammatory bowel disease and psoriasis. Omega-3 is essential for brain function and can reduce the risk of developing Alzheimer's. It is important during pregnancy – DHA in particular is essential for the development of the foetus's brain and eyes. Increasing your intake of omega-3 can help to reduce the risk of heart attack, improve skin and bone

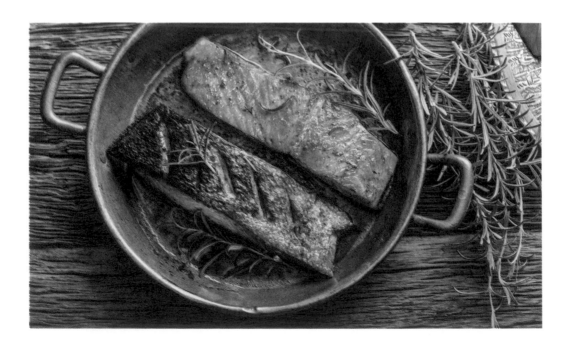

health, and potentially reduce the symptoms of depression.

It is thought that omega-3 effectively reduces inflammation by decreasing the production of inflammatory cytokines and enzymes, as well as releasing resolvins, molecules that help to turn off immune activation and 'resolve' inflammation.

Oily fish to look out for include:

- Anchovies
- Carp
- Eel
- Herring
- Mackerel
- Pilchards
- Salmon
- Sardines
- Sprats
- Trout
- Whitebait

TIP: To help you remember which are oily fish, use the acronym SMASH (salmon, mackerel, anchovies, sardines, herring). This focuses on the oily fish that are most easy to find in shops.

How to use oily fish

- Make a salsa verde with anchovies, fresh herbs, olive oil, garlic, capers and red wine vinegar

- Add anchovies to homemade pizza (*see page 116 for a Cauliflower Pizza recipe*)

- Make mackerel pâté

- Grill whitebait and serve with homemade aioli

- Top a crisp salad with a grilled mackerel fillet

- Use salmon fillets for a tray bake with peppers, tomatoes and sweet potato

- Cook salmon fillets 'en papillote' (wrapped in baking parchment and baked in the oven) with onion, garlic, lemon and parsley

- Enjoy sardines on toast

- Bake trout whole in the oven with lemon, garlic and samphire

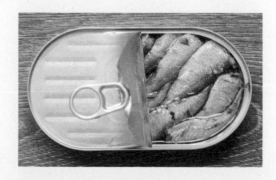

Olive oil

Olive oil is a delicious, versatile and exceptionally healthy addition to your diet. It has an impressive array of over 200 health-promoting components, including a monounsaturated omega-9 fatty acid called oleic acid, polyphenols, cholesterol-lowering phytosterols, a skin-loving compound called squalene and vitamins E and K.

Health benefits of olive oil

Olive oil is a useful tool for heart health – studies show that it can lower blood pressure, prevent plaque build-up in the arteries, reduce 'bad' LDL cholesterol and triglycerides, and increase HDL, the protective form of cholesterol.[17]

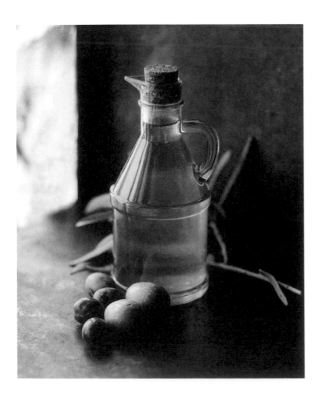

Regular consumption of olive oil can lower blood sugar levels, improve insulin sensitivity[18][19] and, as part of a Mediterranean-style diet, can help to reduce your risk of developing type 2 diabetes by up to 52 per cent.[20][21]

The oleic acid in olive oil can help to protect the brain. This acid is found in abundance in the brain and forms a large part of the myelin sheath, the protective coating surrounding nerve cells. Olive oil has shown promising results in the prevention of Alzheimer's and in reducing the symptoms of depression.

Olive oil has excellent anti-inflammatory properties. One of its phenolic compounds, called oleocanthal, acts on the same pathways as ibuprofen, helping to dampen inflammation and pain. This makes it useful for inflammatory conditions like rheumatoid arthritis.[22]

Olive oil is packed full of antioxidants, which help to protect the body from oxidative stress and reduce the risk of chronic disease. Squalene in particular, can help to protect against skin cancer, so an olive oil-drenched salad while enjoying the sunshine is a particularly wise combination!

How to use olive oil

- Use it to make a salad dressing

- Add to smoothies

- Combine olive oil with egg yolk, lemon juice, apple cider vinegar and mustard to make homemade mayonnaise

- Pour some into a bowl with balsamic vinegar or fresh herbs and use as a dip for fresh bread

- Infuse oil with garlic, fresh herbs or chilli and use on meat, fish or vegetables

- Add to homemade hummus, tzatziki or baba ganoush

- Make crackers with olive oil and chickpea, buckwheat or oat flour

- Pour over steamed vegetables on serving

- Use in mashed potato instead of butter

- Use for casseroles, stews and soups

- Bake a cake using olive oil

- Combine with honey, egg, avocado or coconut oil to make a hair mask

Choosing olive oil

The quality of olive oil is very important. Follow these tips to ensure you're getting the most out of it:

- Look for olive oil that says 'cold pressed' or 'extra virgin' on the label. Avoid any that say 'refined', 'pure', or 'light' (this means the oil is a poor-quality refined oil that lacks the health benefits of cold-pressed oil)

- Olive oil stored in dark glass bottles is best

- Store your olive oil out of direct sunlight and away from heat (in a cool cupboard is ideal, away from your oven or hob)

- Once opened, olive oil stays fresh for one to two months. Buy smaller bottles if you can't use it up in that time

A common misconception is that you can't cook with extra virgin olive oil. Extra virgin olive oil has a reasonably high smoke point, and the high polyphenol content helps to protect the oil from oxidizing, so it's fine for low–medium heat cooking.

Walnuts

The humble walnut is a powerhouse of nutrition, packed full of healthy fats, fibre, vitamins and minerals.

Health benefits of walnuts

It's fascinating how mother nature produces food that looks like the body part it's able to help. Looking at a walnut, you can see how the folds and wrinkles and overall shape look strikingly similar to the human brain. Of all the nuts, walnuts are richest in alpha-linoleic acid, a plant-based form of omega-3. Omega-3 is essential for a healthy brain, and can help to improve cognitive function and reduce inflammation in the brain and nerve cells. There is promising research to suggest that improving your omega-3 levels can help the management of Alzheimer's by preventing the build-up of beta-amyloid plaque in the brain.[23] Walnuts are also rich in polyphenols, which help to protect neurons and suppress brain inflammation.

Walnuts have higher antioxidant levels than any other nut, which comes from vitamin E, melatonin and polyphenols. Melatonin is the hormone that regulates your circadian rhythm (*see page 40*) and possesses potent antioxidant effects. Walnuts contain naturally occurring melatonin, which can help you get a better night's sleep.

Polyphenols feed the beneficial bacteria in your gut. This is useful as having a healthy and abundant gut microflora will help to keep inflammation at bay.

Vitamin E helps to slow the ageing process, prevent hardening of the arteries and keep your skin smooth and supple.

How to make activated nuts

To make nuts easier to digest you can soak them before consuming. Soaking activates the sprouting process and helps to remove phytic acid and enzyme inhibitors, which can hinder mineral absorption and impede digestion.

Add 2 cups of walnuts to a bowl and cover with filtered water and 1 teaspoon of salt. Leave to soak for 5–8 hours. When they're ready, discard the water and rinse the nuts well.

They can be consumed as they are, or you can get a crunchier texture by putting them in a dehydrator or oven on the lowest setting (no higher than 65°C/150°F) for 12–24 hours.

How to use walnuts

- Soak walnuts overnight, rinse, blend with water, then strain through muslin cloth to make fresh walnut milk
- Blend to make walnut butter
- Add chopped walnuts to porridge, salad or yogurt
- Use walnut oil in salad dressing
- Make a trail mix with walnuts, cranberries, pumpkin seeds and cacao nibs
- Try walnut pesto, made with walnuts, basil, garlic, olive oil and salt
- Mix walnuts with desiccated coconut, dates and tahini to make energy balls
- Enjoy sliced apple, walnuts and cheese as a snack
- Bake a spiced raisin and walnut loaf
- Make a walnut and herb crust for fish, meat or roast vegetables
- Whip up vegan meatballs using walnuts, chickpeas, garlic, onion and herbs

TIP: Store your nuts in a glass jar in the fridge to keep them fresh and preserve their nutritional content.

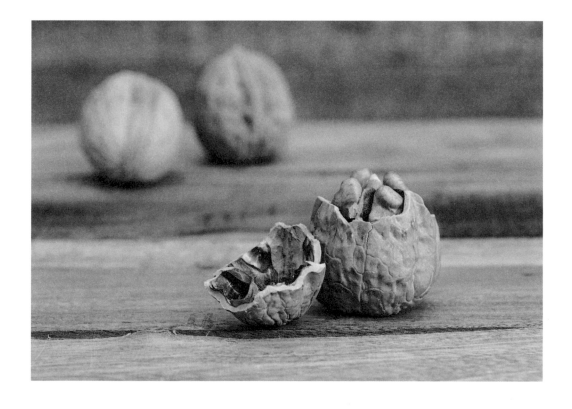

Cruciferous vegetables

These vegetables take their name from the Latin word *cruciferae*, meaning 'cross-bearing', which refers to their cross-shaped flowers. Cruciferous vegetables are quite a large family, including the following:

- Bok choy
- Brussels sprouts
- Cabbage
- Cauliflower
- Daikon
- Horseradish
- Kale
- Kohlrabi
- Mustard
- Radish
- Rapini
- Rocket
- Spinach
- Sprouts
- Swede
- Swiss chard
- Turnip
- Wasabi
- Watercress

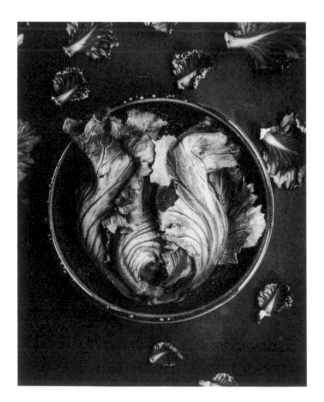

Health benefits of cruciferous vegetables

From a nutritional perspective, cruciferous vegetables really deliver. They are an excellent source of antioxidants, folate, vitamins C, E, K, minerals and fibre. They contain insoluble fibre, which can help to maintain healthy bowel movements and prevent constipation, and soluble fibre, which can help to lower LDL cholesterol, balance blood sugar levels, keep you fuller for longer and feed the beneficial bacteria in your gut.

Cruciferous vegetables are a rich source of sulphoraphane, a sulphur-containing phytochemical with a host of health benefits. Sulphoraphane can help to drive down inflammation by inhibiting NF-kB.

Studies have linked a higher intake of cruciferous vegetables with a significantly reduced risk of cancer.[24] Sulforaphane can help to guard against cancer by supporting the detoxification of carcinogens and inhibiting the growth of cancer cells.[25] By supporting the liver and improving detoxification, it can also guard against damage caused by medication, toxic chemicals and alcohol.

Another exciting compound found in cruciferous vegetables is called indole-3-carbinol. Both indole-3-carbinol (I3C) and one of its metabolites diindolylmethane (DIM) appear to be effective in preventing oestrogen-dependent cancers such as breast, cervical and colon cancer.

How to use cruciferous vegetables

- Grow your own broccoli sprouts and add to salads and smoothies or eat on their own with olive oil and a sprinkle of rock or sea salt

- Make a super greens soup with broccoli, spinach and watercress

- Try a watercress sauce to accompany fish or nut roast

- Make coleslaw with shredded cabbage and carrots

- Steam broccoli and kale, then serve with olive oil and salt

- Add spinach to an omelette

- Use cabbage, broccoli, bok choy and kale in a stir-fry

- Make kale chips with olive oil, salt and nutritional yeast

- Add rocket and sliced radishes to a salad

- Make pesto with spinach or rocket

- Roast cauliflower with olive oil, turmeric, cumin and almonds

- Make latkes or fritters with swede, egg and onion

- Use cauliflower to make mash instead of potatoes

- Make broccoli 'rice' by pulsing in blender until it resembles grains of rice, then bake or soften in a pan with olive oil

- Pan fry cabbage with coconut oil and garlic

Goitrogen concerns

Some people are concerned about the goitrogen content of cruciferous vegetables. Goitrogens can interfere with thyroid function by preventing the uptake of iodine. Realistically you'd have to eat a huge amount to cause a problem, but if you have thyroid issues and you want to be on the safe side, just avoid having lots of green smoothies or juices made with raw cruciferous vegetables. You can lessen any impact by cooking – steaming greatly reduces the level of goitrogens but preserves the nutritional content. Broccoli sprouts don't contain any goitrogens, and are by far the richest source of sulforaphane. They can be grown easily at home in a sprouting tray.

Garlic

Apart from being a delicious ingredient for cooking, garlic has many wonderful health benefits. It has been revered for its medicinal properties for thousands of years.

Health benefits of garlic

Much of garlic's therapeutic effects come from its sulphur-containing compounds, called thiosulphinates, which give garlic its strong flavour and smell. Thiosulphinates have anti-inflammatory and antioxidant activity.

One of the main active components of garlic is a sulphur compound called allicin, which has powerful anti-viral, anti-fungal and antibacterial properties. It is useful for staving off colds and flu, and can help you bounce back more quickly if you fall prey to a winter bug. One study demonstrated that daily intake of garlic could reduce the number of colds by 63 per cent compared to a placebo, and cut recovery time from five to five and a half days for those who did get sick.[26]

Garlic has also shown promise in breaking down biofilms. A biofilm is a slimy, extracellular matrix that bacteria and fungi can form around themselves for protection. Biofilms pose a major challenge to health as our immune systems and drugs have difficulty penetrating them. Without breaking down the biofilm it's very difficult to target an infection. This can lead to chronic, treatment-resistant infections and a huge amount of inflammation.

Garlic is an excellent tool for supporting cardiovascular health. Research suggests that garlic can help to lower harmful forms of cholesterol, reduce blood pressure and prevent hardening of the arteries.

Garlic is perhaps one of the earliest 'performance-enhancing' agents: Olympic athletes in Ancient Greece were given garlic to increase strength and endurance. If you're an athlete or fitness enthusiast, you may want to try it for yourself – research suggests that a regular intake of garlic can help to improve exercise performance, reduce fatigue and promote recovery.[27]

TIP: To get the most out of garlic, it's best to consume it raw. This is because cooking garlic can deactivate an important enzyme called alliinase. If you do want to cook it, a good trick to preserve some of the benefits is to first chop or crush the cloves and leave them to rest for ten minutes before cooking. Chopping or crushing garlic releases the alliinase enzyme, which catalyzes the formation of allicin. Allicin then breaks down to form a variety of beneficial sulphur compounds.

How to use garlic

- If you have a toothache or feel a cold coming on, hold a garlic clove in your mouth, biting down every few minutes to release the garlic juice. Discard the clove after 30 minutes.
- Sauté onion and garlic for soups, casseroles or pasta dishes, then add some raw crushed garlic on serving
- Add to a stir-fry

- Make garlic-infused olive oil
- Make garlic mayonnaise
- Add to dips such as hummus, baba ganoush or tzatziki
- Use garlic in salad dressings
- Perk up sauces such as pesto, salsa verde or chimichurri with garlic
- Roast whole cloves of garlic with peppers, onions and courgettes

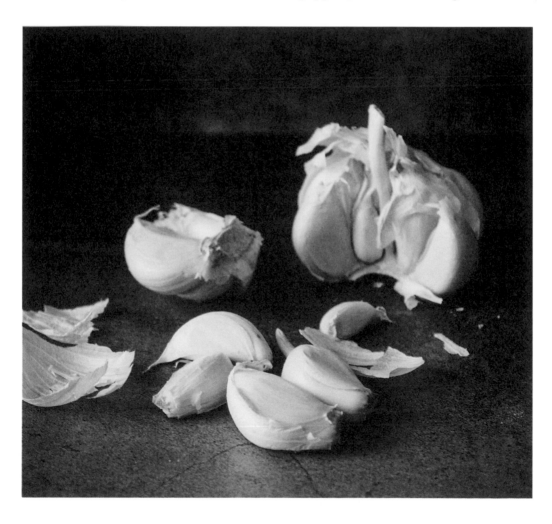

Berries

Berries truly are one of the healthiest foods you can eat. Not only are they sweet, juicy and delicious, but they are one of the best anti-inflammatory tools from mother nature's pharmacy. One of my greatest joys is picking wild blackberries in autumn, and with sticky, purple-stained hands returning the treasure home to make a warming compote.

Health benefits of berries

Berries are loaded with many different types of polyphenols, including anthocyanins, quercetin, resveratrol and ellagic acid. These polyphenols have antioxidant properties to protect the plant from ultraviolet radiation or attack from bacteria. When consumed, our bodies benefit from these antioxidants. The abundance of antioxidants make berries a highly effective tool to help prevent inflammation.

Anthocyanins belong to the flavonoid group of polyphenols and are responsible for the rich purple, red and blue colour of berries. They are known to be one of the most powerful antioxidants. Berries contain a huge amount of anthocyanin compared to other fruits. Anthocyanins have exceptional health-promoting properties, including helping to reduce inflammation, reduce cancer

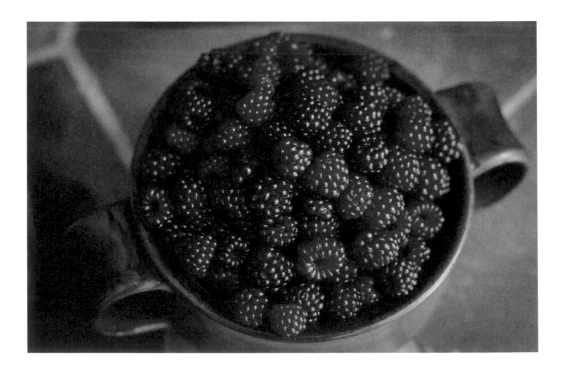

risk, protect against heart disease and cognitive decline, support lung health and prevent urinary tract infections.

Berries are an excellent source of vitamin C. Vitamin C is an essential nutrient and potent antioxidant that can help to support brain and immune function, boost mitochondrial function, protect bones and preserve lung function.

Berries are a good source of soluble fibre, which can slow the absorption of sugar and help you feel fuller for longer. They are lower in sugar than most other fruits and their anthocyanin content helps to improve insulin sensitivity and lower blood glucose levels.[28] This makes berries a great choice for diabetics or those trying to lose weight.

How to use berries

- Add berries to a smoothie

- Use berries to make a warm compote with spices such as cinnamon and nutmeg

- Make a healthy blackberry crumble with a topping made of nuts, desiccated coconut, coconut oil and ground almonds

- Top porridge with berries on serving

- Try an overnight bircher muesli with berries, oats, nuts, seeds and milk of choice

- Add to desserts (*see page 122 for Chia Vanilla Summer Pudding*)

- Make berry sorbet with berries, lemon juice and stevia

- Add fresh berries to yogurt, along with chopped nuts and fresh mint

- Enjoy a handful of berries and nuts as a snack

TIP: To get the most out of berries it's best to consume them raw. Eating them raw means more of the nutrients and phytonutrients will be intact. It's also a good idea to choose organic berries as non-organic berries can contain high amounts of pesticide residue. If this proves too expensive, then a more cost-effective option is to buy bags of frozen berries to add to smoothies, stir into porridge or warm in a pan to make compote. Although heating or freezing can reduce some of the phytonutrients, you'll still be getting many of the benefits. You could also try growing your own; some berries, such as strawberries, raspberries and blackberries, are very easy to cultivate.

Water

Our body is a swimming pool for our organs, with at least 60 per cent of it made up of water. Water is critical to the functioning of every cell in the body and some of its vital functions include the following:

- Water makes up 90 per cent of your blood and helps to carry nutrients and oxygen to cells

- Water helps to regulate your body temperature

- Water lubricates your joints, moistens mucus membranes, bathes your brain and protects your spinal cord

- Water is needed for saliva so that you can swallow and digest your food

- Water helps to flush out waste from the body

- Water lubricates bowel movements and prevents constipation

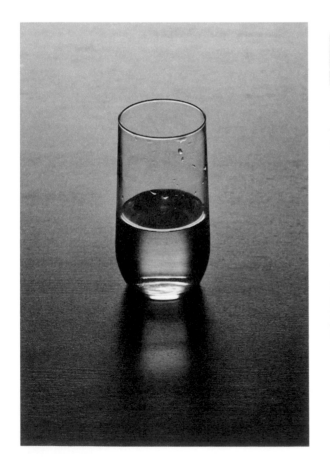

Signs you're not drinking enough water

- You drink coffee, tea or soft drinks more than you drink water
- Dark yellow and strong-smelling urine
- Urinating fewer than four times a day
- Thirst
- Dry skin
- Dizziness
- Headaches
- Brain fog
- Irritability
- Fatigue
- Constipation

Due to the consumption of diuretics (tea, coffee, alcohol and soft drinks), which leach water from the body, and a lack of proper hydration, most people are chronically dehydrated. If the body isn't properly hydrated, it is very difficult for it to function properly.

Dehydration can contribute to chronic inflammation in several ways. If the body doesn't have enough water to detoxify, harmful toxins and cellular waste products can build up in the body and trigger inflammation. A lack of water can reduce the volume of blood and lymphatic fluids, making it harder for immune cells to do their job properly and to protect you from foreign invaders. Dehydration can also impact the delivery of oxygen and essential nutrients to cells, reducing the body's ability to function normally.

How much water should you drink a day?

Aiming for at least 2 litres (3½ pints) of water spread throughout the day is a good starting point. Some people may need more, especially if they are pregnant, or sweating a lot due to exercise or hot weather.

What else can you drink to increase your water intake?

Coffee, tea, alcohol and soft drinks don't count towards your daily water intake as they act as diuretics, causing you to let go of more water than you retain. Better options include soups, broths and vegetable juices, which can both hydrate and supply the body with important nutrients. Herbal teas are also a good choice, or you can enhance the taste of your water by adding fresh mint, cucumber slices or fresh ginger. Filling up a large jug with water at the beginning of the day can be a useful visual aid to help you keep a track of how much you need to drink.

What time of day is best to drink water?

Ideally, spread your water intake throughout the day. Drinking a large glass of water when you wake up is a good way to start the day, as the body is dehydrated after sleep. Avoid drinking large volumes of water with meals as this can impact digestion by diluting the digestive juices. A good rule of thumb is to stop hydrating 30 minutes before a meal, and wait until 60 minutes after food to start again. A few sips of water to lubricate the mouth during meals is fine, but try not to down a pint of water straight after you've finished eating.

A LOOK AT NUTRIENTS

All nutrients work together to promote good health, but certain nutrients are particularly important for keeping inflammation at bay.

Vitamin D

Optimal vitamin D levels are essential for good health, and a deficiency is associated with increased levels of inflammation. Aside from sunlight exposure, we can get vitamin D from oily fish, beef liver, eggs and shiitake mushrooms. If your levels are adequate, but you want to stay topped up, a good maintenance dose is between 500–2000 iu daily. If you are deficient you will likely need much more, so it's wise to get your levels tested regularly. When purchasing a supplement, look for one that contains both vitamins D3 and K2 as they work synergistically together.

Omega-3

Good omega-3 status is one of the best protections against inflammation. The best sources are oily fish, seafood and pastured eggs. Aim to eat oily fish three times a week, and pastured eggs as regularly as you like. For plant sources, focus on walnuts, chia and hemp seeds and flaxseeds.

Cod liver oil is a great source of omega-3 as well as a wealth of other nutrients that can help to reduce inflammation, including vitamins A and D. For people who struggle to eat enough oily fish or are prone to vitamin D deficiency, 1–2 teaspoons per day can be supportive, especially during the winter months. For vegans, a good option is algae oil, but avoid brands that use carrageenan as it has been linked with colon inflammation.

Vitamin C

A potent antioxidant that can help to protect cells from free-radical damage, vitamin C can also increase your levels of glutathione, one the body's most important antioxidants. Vitamin C-rich foods include berries, citrus fruits, asparagus, cruciferous vegetables, peppers, tomatoes and parsley. Many people are deficient, so supplementing with 1000mg a day can be useful to support your immune system.

B vitamins

B vitamins are important for many different functions in the body, including energy production and maintaining the health of the nervous system.

B6 deficiency is associated with an increase in inflammatory markers, while deficiencies in B6, B9 (folate) and B12 are associated with elevated homocysteine, which can significantly increase the risk for heart disease. B6 is found in meat, fish, chicken, peppers, garlic and cruciferous vegetables. B9 is found in leafy green vegetables, nuts, lentils, beans and parsley. B12 is found in meat, chicken, fish, seafood and eggs.

A good-quality B complex can be a good way to top up your levels:
- B6 – look for good doses between 45–50mg
- B9 – look for natural folate (may be listed as folinic acid or methylfolate) rather than folic acid
- B12 – look for methylcobalamin or hydroxocobalamin rather than cyanocobalamin

Magnesium
Magnesium is one of the most important nutrients in our diet, and many people are deficient. It is needed for over 300 chemical reactions in the body and is essential for muscle and nerve function, blood pressure regulation, energy production, balanced blood sugar levels and reducing inflammation. Magnesium is found in many foods, including leafy green vegetables, squash, pumpkin seeds, nuts, grains and legumes.

If topping up with a supplement, look for the more bioavailable forms of magnesium, such as glycinate or citrate. You can also top up your magnesium levels by taking Epsom salts baths, which contain magnesium sulphate.

Supplements: can you get what you need from food?

The foundation of your anti-inflammatory strategy should be good food. No supplement can remedy the harmful effects of a poor diet, nor can it replicate the magical synergy of nutritional compounds, enzymes and cofactors that are found in food. However, certain factors can make it difficult to meet all nutritional needs through food alone. Modern intensive agricultural methods have led to soil becoming increasingly depleted of nutrients, while many of us have a greater need for nutritional support due to stress, less time outdoors and increased exposure to food and environmental toxins. Certain supplements, such as the B vitamins opposite, can help keep inflammation at bay.

Sub-standard supplements, however, tend to contain long lists of unnecessary excipients, such as bulking agents, fillers and preservatives, as well as synthetic forms of nutrients that can have harmful effects. Invest in good-quality supplements that contain the most natural and bioavailable forms of nutrients.

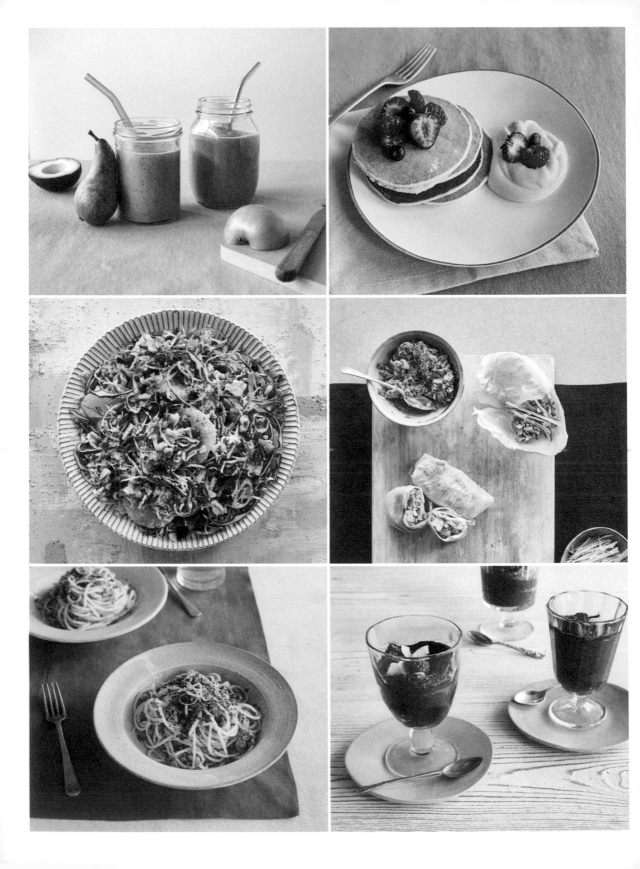

4

RECIPES

A healthy balanced diet is an important part of keeping yourself well and keeping inflammation in check. This chapter includes 30 mouthwatering recipes, each one featuring an array of powerful anti-inflammatory ingredients, nicely balanced with protein, complex carbohydrates, healthy fats and fibre to keep your blood sugar levels stable. There are recipes for breakfast, lunch, dinner, snacks and healthy sweet treats, all chosen because they include the key nutrients needed to prevent inflammation and promote health and vitality.

TURMERIC AND COCONUT MILK LATTE

SERVES 1 | **PREP:** 5 minutes | **COOK:** 5–10 minutes

Commonly known as 'golden milk', this warmly spiced latte provides a comforting 'hug in a mug' at any time of day, not just breakfast. Turmeric and ginger have powerful anti-inflammatory properties and are great for supporting digestion. Reduced-fat canned coconut milk is used but you can use full-fat if you want a creamier latte.

250ml (8½fl oz) reduced-fat coconut milk
1 tsp ground turmeric
1 tsp finely grated root ginger
freshly ground black pepper
1 cinnamon stick
2 cardamom pods, crushed
pinch of nutmeg
stevia, to taste

Tip: Adding 1 teaspoon coconut oil will make it easier for your body to absorb the turmeric.

Variations:

• Unsweetened almond milk can be substituted for the coconut milk.
• Add the scraped-out seeds of ½ vanilla pod.
• Make the latte spicier by adding a pinch of cayenne pepper.
• Add a star anise or a pinch of Chinese 5-spice powder.

1 Whisk together the coconut milk, turmeric, ginger and black pepper until well combined and frothy.

2 Transfer to a saucepan and add the cinnamon stick and crushed cardamom pods. Bring to the boil, then reduce heat and cook gently over a low to medium heat until just simmering. Simmer for 5 minutes, whisking once or twice.

3 Remove from the heat and sweeten to taste with stevia. Strain through a sieve or fine mesh strainer into a mug.

BERRY AND MINT SMOOTHIE

SERVES 2 | **PREP:** 10 minutes

Berries are low in sugar compared to other fruits and packed with inflammation-fighting antioxidants. Surprisingly filling, this smoothie is a healthy way to kickstart your day or enjoy as a healthy snack.

240ml (8fl oz) non-dairy kefir

120ml (4fl oz) almond milk

1 tbsp almond butter

115g (4oz) frozen mixed berries, such as strawberries, raspberries, blueberries

100g (3½oz) ripe cherries, stoned

1 frozen banana

juice of 1 large orange

a small handful of fresh mint

stevia, to sweeten

coconut flakes, for sprinkling

Tip: Keep a pack of frozen berries handy in your freezer to use all year round.

Variations:

- Substitute coconut milk for the almond milk, or dairy-free yogurt for the kefir, or use goat's milk kefir.
- Add a teaspoon of ground turmeric for an anti-inflammatory boost.
- Use fresh berries instead of frozen.

1 Put the kefir, almond milk, almond butter and fruit in a blender or food processor. Add the orange juice and most of the mint, reserving a few small sprigs.

2 Blitz until the smoothie is thick, creamy and smooth. If it's too thick for your liking, thin it with a little almond milk or water until you get the desired consistency.

3 Sweeten to taste with stevia and divide between 2 tall glasses or shallow bowls (for a smoothie bowl). Decorate with the reserved mint and sprinkle with coconut flakes. Serve immediately.

AVOCADO MATCHA SMOOTHIE

SERVES 4 | **PREP:** 15 minutes

This smoothie is packed with goodness, including nutrient-dense leafy greens, antioxidant-rich matcha green tea powder and avocado and coconut milk to give you a dose of healthy fats.

1 ripe avocado, peeled and stoned

50g (2oz) kale or spinach, trimmed, washed and shredded

2 green dessert apples, cored and chopped

1 pear, cored and chopped

750ml (1¼ pints) coconut milk

4 tbsp dairy-free coconut yogurt

2 tsp matcha powder

a few ice cubes (optional)

1 Put the avocado, kale or spinach, apples, pear, coconut milk, yogurt and matcha powder in a powerful blender. Add ice cubes.

2 Blitz until well blended, creamy and smooth.

3 Pour into 4 tall glasses and serve immediately.

....

Tip: Make this smoothie at the last minute to enjoy the vibrant green colour. Avocados can discolour quickly after they are cut open.

....

Variations:

• Add a good dash of lime or lemon juice for extra vitamin C and a sharp citrus flavour.

• For a thicker smoothie, add a large sliced banana.

• Substitute unsweetened almond milk for the coconut milk.

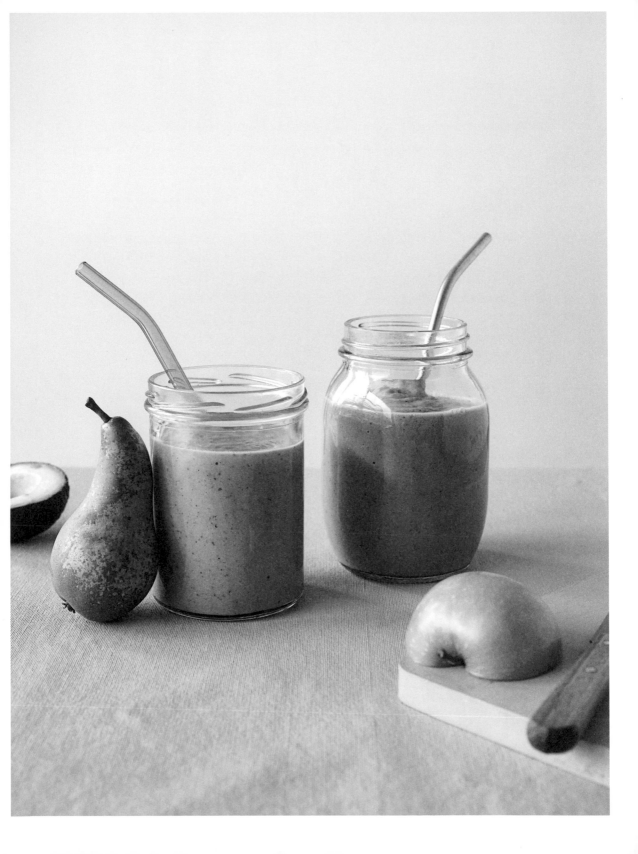

BLUEBERRY OVERNIGHT OATS

SERVES 4 | **PREP:** 10 minutes | **CHILL:** overnight

A quick breakfast, it takes only 10 minutes to prepare these delicious overnight oats the night before. Just pop them into the fridge and top with fruit the next morning. With a low glycaemic index, oats will make you feel full for longer so you're less likely to snack before lunch.

200g (7oz) rolled or porridge oats

500ml (18fl oz) unsweetened almond milk

400g (14oz) dairy-free yogurt

2 tbsp chia seeds

2-3 drops vanilla extract

2 tbsp mixed seeds, such as flax and
   sunflower

4 tbsp chopped almonds or walnuts

200g (7oz) fresh blueberries

Tip: Use frozen instead of fresh fruit and place on top of the oat and milk mixture before chilling. The juices will add flavour and colour.

Variations:

- Try different fruit toppings, such as raspberries, strawberries and cherries, or even some sliced banana.
- If you have a sweet tooth, add some stevia to taste to the oat and milk mixture.
- Use coconut milk instead of almond milk.
- Instead of vanilla, flavour with grated orange zest.

1 Put the oats, milk, yogurt and chia seeds in a bowl and mix together well. Add vanilla extract to taste.

2 Divide the mixture between 4 glass screw-top jars. Sprinkle the mixed seeds and nuts over the top. Cover with the lids or cling film and chill in the fridge overnight, preferably for at least 8 hours, so the oats and chia seeds can absorb all the liquid.

3 The following morning, remove from the fridge and top with the blueberries. Eat immediately.

HAZELNUT PORRIDGE WITH RHUBARB

SERVES 4 | **PREP:** 10 minutes | **COOK:** 15 minutes

Oats are high in fibre, rich in nutrients and contain prebiotics that support your gut flora, all of which can help to lower inflammation in your body. This porridge is topped with rhubarb cooked with ginger and orange juice.

1kg (2lb 4oz) young pink rhubarb, trimmed and cut into chunks

2.5cm (1in) fresh root ginger, peeled and grated

grated zest and juice of 1 orange

stevia, to taste (optional)

60g (2oz) hazelnuts

225g (8oz) rolled porridge oats

1.2 litres (2 pints) unsweetened almond milk

a pinch of sea salt

115g (4oz) dairy-free coconut yogurt

....

Variations:

- Substitute a tangerine, satsuma, clementine or mandarin for the orange.
- Add a cinnamon stick to the rhubarb.
- Use walnuts or almonds instead of the hazelnuts.
- If rhubarb is not in season, top with berries instead.

1 Preheat the oven to 200°C (180°C fan/400°F/Gas 6).

2 Place the rhubarb in a large ovenproof dish and sprinkle with the ginger and orange zest. Pour the orange juice over the top and cook in the preheated oven for 15 minutes or until just tender. Don't overcook or it will go mushy – you want it to keep its shape. If wished, sweeten to taste with stevia.

3 At the same time, spread the hazelnuts in a single layer on a baking tray and toast in the oven, above the rhubarb, for 10–15 minutes until golden brown and fragrant. Remove and wrap in a clean tea towel for 1 minute, then rub the nuts vigorously to remove the skins. Cool and chop coarsely.

4 Put the oats and almond milk in a saucepan. Add the salt and stir over a medium to high heat until it comes to the boil. Reduce to a simmer, stirring occasionally, for 5 minutes until smooth.

5 Divide between 4 shallow serving bowls and top with the rhubarb, yogurt and toasted hazelnuts.

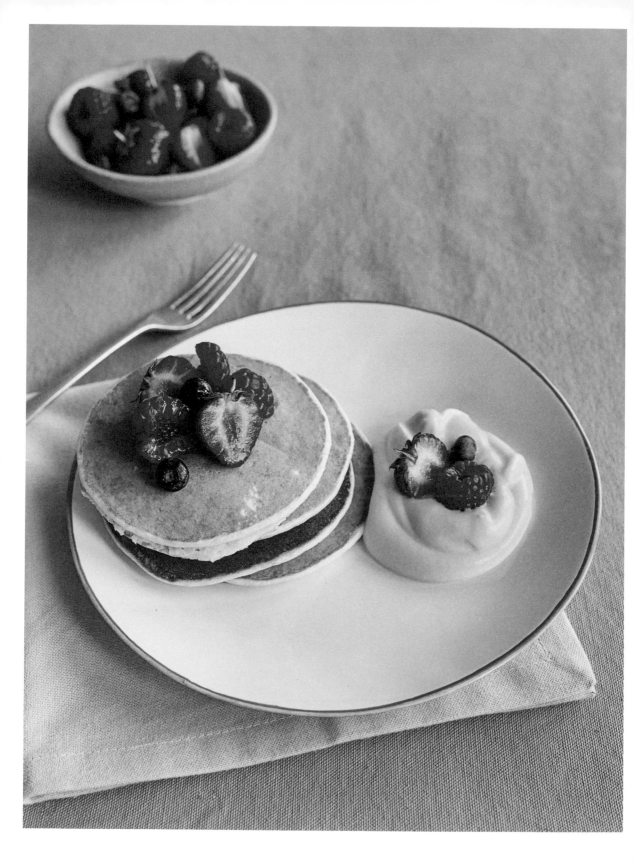

BUCKWHEAT BREAKFAST PANCAKES

SERVES 4 | **PREP:** 10 minutes | **COOK:** 10–15 minutes

These light and fluffy breakfast pancakes are free from sugar, gluten and dairy, and make a crowd-pleasing breakfast. They won't spike blood sugar levels like traditional pancakes made with refined flour and sugar.

2 large organic free-range eggs

220ml (7½fl oz) unsweetened almond milk

5 tbsp light olive oil, plus extra for cooking

1 tsp vanilla extract

100g (3½oz) buckwheat flour

100g (3½oz) gluten-free plain flour

2 tsp gluten-free baking powder

1 tsp ground cinnamon

½ tsp salt

a pinch of stevia (optional)

dairy-free coconut yogurt, to serve

mixed berries, such as blueberries, raspberries, strawberries, to serve

....

Variations:

- Sprinkle shredded coconut on top of the pancakes, to serve.
- Serve with juicy dark cherries or sliced bananas, instead of berries.

1 In a bowl, beat the eggs, almond milk, olive oil and vanilla extract until well blended.

2 Sift the flours, baking powder and cinnamon in a large bowl. Stir in the salt and stevia and make a well in the centre. Pour in the beaten egg mixture and whisk until everything is well combined.

3 Set a large non-stick frying pan or griddle over a medium to high heat and lightly brush with oil. When it's really hot, drop a few tablespoons of batter into the pan, leaving plenty of space in between. When bubbles appear on the surface, after 1–2 minutes, flip the pancakes over and cook for 1–2 minutes more until set and browned. Remove and keep warm while you make the rest in the same way.

4 Serve the pancakes hot, topped with a large spoonful of dairy-free yogurt and the berries.

TURMERIC SCRAMBLED EGGS

SERVES 4 | **PREP:** 5 minutes | **COOK:** 12–15 minutes

Upgrade your usual breakfast eggs by including turmeric and spinach, both of which have excellent anti-inflammatory properties.

8 large organic free-range eggs
4 tbsp coconut milk
2 tsp ground turmeric or 2 tbsp grated fresh root
1 tsp coconut oil
1 garlic clove, crushed
200g (7oz) baby spinach leaves
salt and freshly ground black pepper
toasted gluten-free bread, to serve

....

Variations:
- Cook a thinly sliced spring onion with the garlic.
- For a spicier version, add a finely diced bird's-eye chilli.
- Make herby eggs by adding chopped coriander, flat-leaf parsley or chives.

1 Break the eggs into a bowl and add the coconut milk, turmeric and salt and pepper. Beat together until well combined.

2 Heat the coconut oil in a non-stick pan set over a medium heat. When it melts, add the garlic and cook, stirring, for 1 minute without browning. Tip in the spinach and cook for 2–3 minutes until it wilts and turns bright green.

3 Reduce the heat to low and add the beaten egg mixture. Stir gently with a wooden spoon, pulling the cooked edges in from the sides, until the scrambled eggs start to thicken and are softly set and creamy. Take your time and be patient – they may take 6–8 minutes to scramble. Be careful not to overcook them – the mixture should not colour and turn brown and crisp underneath.

4 Serve immediately with the gluten-free toast.

GREEN BREAKFAST FRITTERS

SERVES 4 | **PREP:** 25 minutes | **COOK:** 12–15 minutes

Packed full of greens, these tasty vegetable fritters are really quick and easy to make for a delicious breakfast or weekend brunch. Green vegetables are an important part of an anti-inflammatory diet.

400g (14oz) courgettes, trimmed
200g (7oz) broccoli florets, finely chopped
a large handful of baby spinach leaves, coarsely shredded
a bunch of fresh flat-leaf parsley, chopped
3 large organic free-range eggs
grated zest of 1 lemon
4 tbsp chickpea (gram) flour
salt and freshly ground black pepper
olive oil for frying

Tzatziki:

400g (14oz) thick dairy-free yogurt
1 small cucumber, peeled and diced
2 garlic cloves, crushed
a handful of fresh mint, finely chopped
a handful of fresh dill, finely chopped
juice of ½ lemon
1 tsp white wine vinegar
salt and freshly ground black pepper

Tip: You can prepare the tzatziki the day before and chill it in the fridge overnight.

Variations:

• Substitute spring greens for spinach.
• Vary the herbs – include snipped chives, dried oregano or mint.

1 Make the tzatziki: mix all the ingredients together in a bowl and season to taste with salt and pepper. Cover and chill in the fridge while you make the fritters.

2 Grate the courgettes coarsely into a bowl, squeezing out any excess moisture with your hands. Add the broccoli, spinach and herbs.

3 In a clean, dry bowl, beat the eggs and then mix in the vegetables, herbs and lemon zest. Gently stir in the flour and seasoning to taste.

4 Add a little olive oil to a non-stick frying pan and set over a medium heat. When the pan is hot, add 2 –3 serving spoons of the vegetable batter, one at a time, so they have room around them to spread out.

5 Cook for 2–3 minutes until golden brown and set underneath. Flip the fritters over and cook the other side. Remove from the pan, drain on kitchen paper and keep warm while you cook the remaining fritters in the same way.

6 Serve the fritters immediately while they're piping hot with the chilled tzatziki on the side.

SMOKY SPICED ROASTED CHICKPEAS

MAKES approx. 500g (1lb 2oz) | **PREP:** 10 minutes | **COOK:** 25–35 minutes

Roasted chickpeas make a delicious, healthy snack that is high in protein. Rather than soaking dried chickpeas and cooking them from scratch, canned are used here for convenience. The roasted chickpeas also add crunch to salads and rice bowls.

2 x 400g (14oz) cans chickpeas, drained and rinsed

2 tbsp olive oil

½ tsp fine sea salt

1 tsp smoked paprika

½ tsp ground cumin seeds

½ tsp ground ginger

a pinch each of ground cinnamon and cayenne pepper

....

Tip: You don't need to use expensive extra-virgin olive oil - any olive oil will work well, as the spices provide the flavour.

....

Variations:

- For a touch of heat, add a little chilli powder.
- Add garlic powder and dried oregano or thyme.

1 Preheat the oven to 200°C (180°C fan/400°F/Gas 6).

2 Put the chickpeas in a bowl with the olive oil and sea salt and stir gently. Add the paprika, cumin seeds, ground spices and cayenne and toss lightly until the chickpeas are evenly coated.

3 Spread them out in a single layer on a baking tray. Roast in the preheated oven for 25–35 minutes, turning them over after 15 minutes, until crisp and golden brown. Check them towards the end of the cooking time to make sure they don't catch and burn.

4 Remove from the oven and leave to cool on the tray. Store in a sealed container or plastic bag at room temperature for 2-3 days.

ROASTED SQUASH AND LENTIL SALAD

SERVES 4 | **PREP:** 20 minutes | **COOK:** 30–35 minutes

Lentils are a great source of plant protein, dietary fibre, B vitamins and zinc. If you can't get Puy lentils, any green or brown lentils will work well, but avoid the little red ones, which can become mushy when cooked.

450g (1lb) butternut squash, peeled, deseeded and cubed

2 red peppers, deseeded and diced

6 tbsp olive oil

200g (7oz) Puy lentils (dried weight), rinsed

1 large red onion, chopped

2 large carrots, diced

2 celery sticks, diced

2 garlic cloves, crushed

200g (7oz) cherry or baby plum tomatoes, halved (optional)

100g (3½oz) baby spinach leave

a bunch of fresh flat-leaf parsley, chopped

juice of 1 lemon

balsamic vinegar for drizzling

salt and freshly ground black pepper

Tip: If you're in a hurry, use canned lentils or the variety you buy in pouches and microwave instead of dried lentils.

Variations:

- Top the salad with roasted pumpkin, red onions, carrots, courgettes or fennel.
- Vary the herbs: try coriander, dill or mint.
- Serve with thinly sliced smoked salmon.

1 Preheat the oven to 200°C (180°C fan/400°F/Gas 6).

2 Place the squash and red pepper in a large roasting pan. Drizzle with 3 tablespoons of olive oil and season. Roast for 30–35 minutes, turning occasionally, until golden brown.

3 Meanwhile, put the lentils in a pan and cover with cold water. Bring to the boil, then reduce the heat and simmer gently for 15–20 minutes, until they are cooked but still retain a little 'bite'. Drain well.

4 While the lentils are simmering, heat the remaining olive oil in a large frying pan and cook the red onion, carrots, celery and garlic over a low to medium heat, stirring, for 8–10 minutes until softened.

5 Stir the lentils into the onion mixture, and add the tomatoes (if using), spinach and most of the parsley. Heat through gently, then stir in the lemon juice and vinegar. Season and remove from the heat.

6 Transfer to 4 bowls, top with the roasted vegetables, sprinkle over parsley and drizzle with balsamic. Serve at room temperature.

RAINBOW SLAW

SERVES 4–6 | **PREP:** 20 minutes

This crunchy slaw is a great winter salad and provides an abundance of delicious anti-inflammatory ingredients. You can also use it as a side dish with griddled chicken or burgers, as a topping for baked jacket potatoes or as a filling for stuffed vegetables.

200g (7oz) fresh green Brussels sprouts, trimmed and shredded

½ red cabbage, cored and shredded

2 carrots, coarsely grated

1 small red onion, grated

a bunch of fresh flat-leaf parsley, chopped

2 oranges

seeds of 1 pomegranate

100g (3½oz) walnuts, chopped

salt and freshly ground black pepper

Dressing:

4 tbsp extra virgin olive oil

1 tbsp cider vinegar

juice of 1 small orange

1cm (½in) piece fresh root ginger, peeled and grated

1 Mix together the sprouts, red cabbage, carrots, onion and parsley in a large bowl.

2 Cut the peel and all the white pith off the oranges. Slice them horizontally into rounds and then cut into smaller pieces. Add to the salad along with any juice. Stir in the pomegranate seeds and walnuts.

3 Put all the dressing ingredients in a jug or small bowl and whisk until well combined. Pour over the salad and toss gently. Season with salt and pepper.

Tip: For more crunch and an aniseed flavour, add thinly sliced fennel bulb.

Variations:

• Use clementines, satsumas, mandarins or blood oranges instead of oranges.

• Add sunflower, pumpkin, fennel or toasted black mustard seeds.

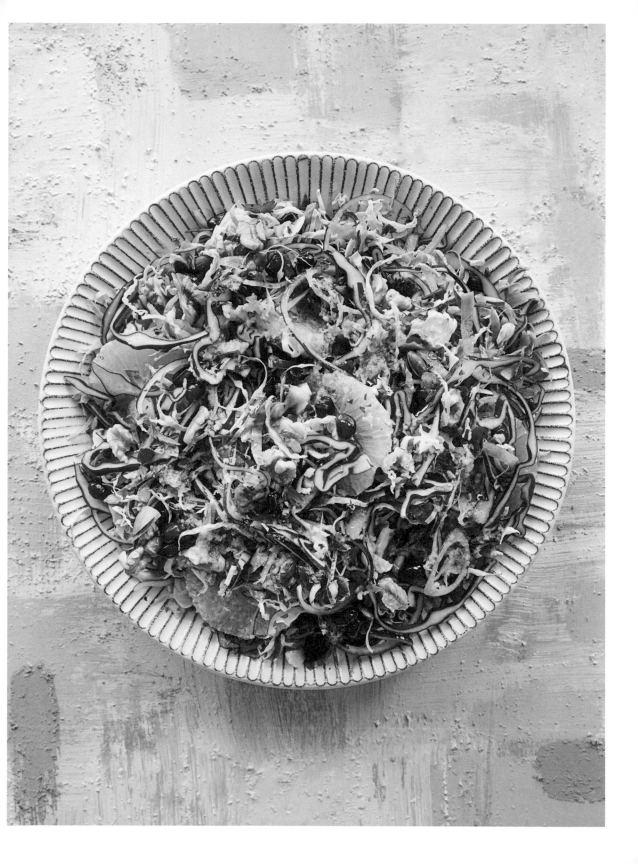

ITALIAN BROCCOLI SALAD

SERVES 4 | **PREP:** 20 minutes | **COOK:** 20 minutes

Broccoli is a versatile vegetable; here it is roasted and made into the star ingredient in a winter salad. One of the healthiest foods, it is high in fibre and an excellent source of vitamins C, E, K and folate.

1 large head broccoli (calabrese)

75ml (3fl oz) olive oil

250g (9oz) stale gluten-free bread, cut into 2cm (¾in) cubes

100g (3½oz) toasted hazelnuts (see page 91)

2 garlic cloves, crushed

grated zest and juice of 1 small lemon

1 tbsp red wine vinegar

1 red bird's eye chilli, deseeded and diced

350g (12oz) cherry or baby plum tomatoes, halved or quartered

1 ripe avocado, peeled, stoned and cubed

6 anchovy fillets in olive oil, drained and chopped

a small bunch of fresh basil, shredded

sea salt crystals and freshly ground black pepper

....

Variations:

• Substitute walnuts or almonds for the hazelnuts.

• Use purple sprouting or tenderstem broccoli instead of calabrese.

• Experiment with different herbs: try chives, mint or parsley.

• Add some thinly sliced spring onions.

1 Preheat the oven to 200°C (180°C fan/400°F/Gas 6).

2 Separate the broccoli florets and slice the stem. Place in a roasting pan and drizzle with 2 tablespoons olive oil. Season lightly with salt and pepper, and place in the preheated oven.

3 After 10 minutes, add the bread cubes to the pan, turning them in the oil. If necessary, drizzle with a little more oil to coat them completely. Bake for a further 10 minutes or until the broccoli is just tender and starting to char and the bread croûtons are crisp and golden.

4 Crush the hazelnuts, garlic and a good pinch of salt in a pestle and mortar. Stir in the remaining olive oil, lemon zest and juice, vinegar and chilli.

5 Put the roasted broccoli and croûtons in a large bowl with the tomatoes, avocado and anchovies. Toss lightly with the basil in the nutty dressing, then season to taste with salt and pepper. Serve immediately while the broccoli is still warm.

QUINOA TABBOULEH WITH RADICCHIO

SERVES 4 | **PREP:** 15 minutes | **COOK:** 20 minutes

Traditionally made with bulgur wheat, this tabbouleh uses gluten-free quinoa instead and is served with griddled radicchio. For the best results, choose a really good-quality flavourful vegetable stock.

200g (7oz) quinoa (dry weight)

480ml (16fl oz) vegetable stock

a bunch of spring onions, finely chopped

225g (8oz) ripe baby plum tomatoes, diced

1 small cucumber, diced

a bunch of fresh flat-leaf parsley, finely chopped

a handful of fresh mint, finely chopped

1–2 garlic cloves, crushed

juice of 2 lemons

5 tbsp fruity green olive oil, plus extra for oiling

60g (2oz) hazelnuts

4 small radicchio heads, cut in half or quarters lengthwise

salt and freshly ground black pepper

seeds of ½ pomegranate

....

Tip: You will know when the quinoa is cooked because the 'sprout' or 'tail' will pop out of the seed.

....

Variations:

• Substitute red or white chicory (Belgian endive) for the radicchio.

• Use toasted pine nuts or seeds instead of hazelnuts.

• Add rocket, watercress or more herbs.

1 Rinse the quinoa under running cold water, then drain. Heat the stock in a large pan and as soon as it starts to boil, tip in the quinoa. Reduce the heat, cover the pan and simmer gently for 15 minutes.

2 Turn off the heat and leave to steam in the pan for 6–8 minutes before draining off any excess liquid. Fluff with a fork and transfer to a bowl.

3 Add the spring onions, tomatoes, herbs, garlic, lemon juice and olive oil. Season to taste and set aside.

4 While the quinoa is cooking, set a dry frying pan over a medium heat and when hot, add the hazelnuts and toast for 1–2 minutes, stirring frequently, until golden brown – don't let them burn. Remove immediately and set aside to cool.

5 Just before serving, lightly oil a ridged griddle pan and set over a medium heat. Add the radicchio and cook for 1–2 minutes until it starts to wilt and slightly char.

6 Divide the tabbouleh between 4 serving plates and top with the radicchio, toasted hazelnuts and pomegranate seeds.

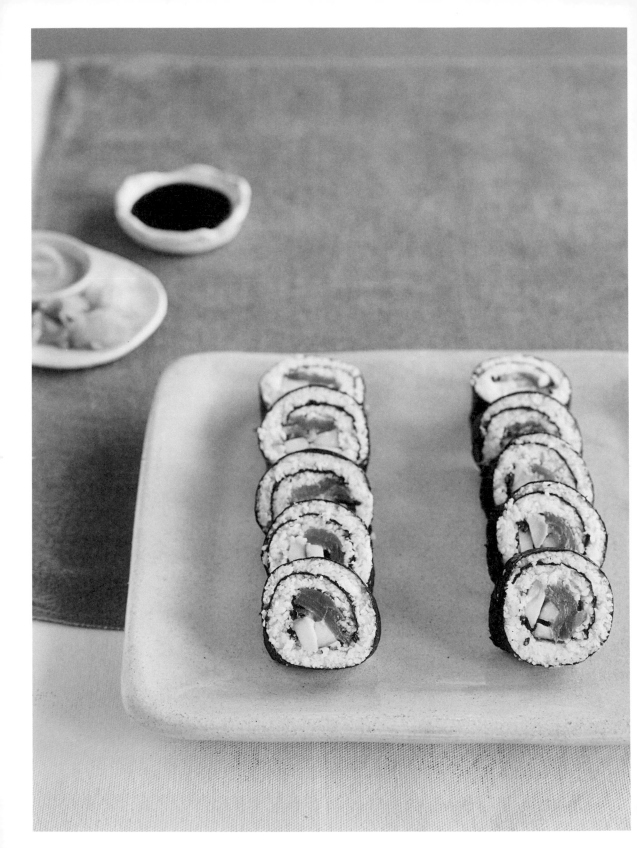

CAULI 'RICE' SUSHI

SERVES 4 | **PREP:** 30 minutes | **COOK:** 3–4 minutes | **CHILL:** 30 minutes

Replacing white rice with cauliflower makes this sushi a low-carbohydrate option that prevents spikes in blood sugar. The smoked salmon is rich in omega-3 fatty acids, while the avocado provides antioxidants.

1 medium cauliflower (approx. 550g/
   1lb 4oz), stem and leaves removed
2 tbsp rice vinegar
1 tsp mirin
sea salt
4 nori sheets
115g (4oz) thinly sliced organic or wild
   smoked salmon, cut into long thin strips
1 tsp wasabi paste
¼ cucumber, peeled, deseeded and cut into
   long thin strips
1 avocado, peeled, stoned and cut into
   long thin strips
1 tbsp black sesame seeds
pickled ginger and gluten-free tamari,
   to serve

Tip: If you don't have a sushi mat, use a work surface covered with cling film.

Variations:

• Serve with gluten-free hot sauce instead of tamari.
• Vegetarians can use blanched thin asparagus spears or cooked sweet potato or squash instead of salmon.

1 Separate the cauliflower into florets and pulse in a food processor until you have rice-sized 'grains'.
2 Place in a glass bowl and cover with cling film. Microwave on high for 3–4 minutes. Spoon the cauliflower onto kitchen paper or a clean tea towel and press out any liquid.
3 Transfer to a bowl and stir in the rice vinegar and mirin.
4 Place the nori sheets, shiny side down, on a sushi mat. Divide the 'rice' between the sheets, spreading it evenly and pressing down with the back of a spoon. Leave a 1cm (½in) border along the long edges.
5 Place the smoked salmon on top and dot with wasabi paste. Top with the cucumber and avocado, then sprinkle with sesame seeds. Using the sushi mat, lift the long bottom edge of each nori sheet over the filling and roll towards the top, pressing down firmly. At the end, brush lightly with water to seal.
6 Put the sushi rolls in the fridge and chill for at least 30 minutes.
7 Cut the sushi rolls into 2.5cm (1in) thick slices and serve.

MEDITERRANEAN FISH SOUP

SERVES 6 | **PREP:** 20 minutes | **COOK:** 45–50 minutes

This hearty fish soup is served throughout the Mediterranean. The ingredients vary according to what is available and in season. Consuming omega-3 fats is an important means of suppressing inflammation.

1kg (2lb 4oz) mixed fish, such as monkfish, cod, hake, sea bream, sea bass, red or grey mullet, whiting, anchovies, sardines, preferably left whole and scaled, cleaned and gutted

4 tbsp fruity olive oil, plus extra for drizzling

1 large onion, chopped

1 fennel bulb, thinly sliced

2 carrots, cut into chunks

2 celery sticks, sliced

3 garlic cloves, crushed

2 courgettes, sliced or cut into matchsticks

500g (1lb 2oz) potatoes, peeled and cubed

450g (1lb) juicy tomatoes, roughly chopped

a pinch of crushed chilli flakes (optional)

1.2 litres (2 pints) good-quality fish stock

a pinch of saffron threads

3 bay leaves

2 strips orange zest

juice of 1 orange or lemon

400g (14oz) spinach or spring greens, washed, trimmed and shredded

salt and freshly ground black pepper

a bunch of fresh flat-leaf parsley, chopped

a small bunch of fresh dill, chopped

Variation:
• Add prawns, mussels, clams or lobster.

1 Rinse the fish under cold running water. Pat dry with kitchen paper and cut the larger ones through the bone into several thick pieces.

2 Heat the olive oil in a large saucepan set over a low to medium heat and cook the onion, fennel, carrots, celery and garlic, stirring, for 10 minutes, or until softened.

3 Add the courgettes, potatoes and tomatoes with the chilli flakes (if using). Stir gently and then add the stock, saffron, bay and orange zest.

4 Bring to the boil, then reduce the heat to a bare simmer and cover the pan. Cook gently for 15–20 minutes, until the vegetables are tender, then add the fish and simmer for a further 10–15 minutes until it is opaque and starting to come away from the bone. Add the orange or lemon juice and the spinach or greens. Cook for 2–3 minutes until they wilt and are tender. Season.

5 Stir in the chopped herbs and ladle the soup into shallow bowls, dividing the fish equally between them. Drizzle with a little olive oil and serve.

CHICKEN AND MUSHROOM MISO

SERVES 4 | **PREP:** 15 minutes | **COOK:** 25 minutes

Use the best-quality stock you can find – or, better still, make your own. It will make all the difference to the flavour of this healthy, cleansing soup. The miso is rich with anti-inflammatory ingredients: ginger, leafy green vegetables, mushrooms, organic chicken and miso paste.

3 tbsp olive oil

8 spring onions, sliced

2 garlic cloves, crushed

1 tbsp finely chopped fresh root ginger

1 celery stick, diced

1 red chilli, deseeded and diced (optional)

300g (10oz) skinned organic chicken breast fillets, thinly sliced

300g (10oz) chestnut mushrooms, sliced

1 litre (33fl oz) hot chicken or vegetable stock

4 tbsp white miso paste

250g (9oz) spring greens or spinach, washed, trimmed and shredded

a dash of lime juice

1-2 tbsp tamari or gluten-free soy sauce

....

Tip: Add 1 teaspoon of rice vinegar at the end of cooking for a hot-and-sour version.

....

Variations:

- Use shiitake mushrooms instead of chestnut mushrooms.
- Substitute kale or dark green cabbage for the spinach or spring greens.
- Add a handful of beansprouts and some chopped fresh coriander.

1 Heat the oil in a large saucepan set over a medium heat. Cook the spring onions, garlic, ginger, celery, chilli, chicken and mushrooms, stirring occasionally, for 6–8 minutes, or until the vegetables soften and the chicken is golden brown.

2 Add the hot stock and bring to the boil. Reduce the heat to a simmer and stir in the miso paste. Keep stirring until it dissolves.

3 Cook gently for 10 minutes, then add the spring greens or spinach and cook for 5 minutes or until the chicken is cooked right through. Stir in the lime juice and tamari to taste.

4 Ladle the hot soup into 4 shallow bowls and serve piping hot.

CARROT AND SWEET POTATO SOUP

SERVES 4 | **PREP:** 20 minutes | **COOK:** 30–35 minutes

This gloriously orange soup is warming and sustaining on a cold day. For a finishing touch, chilli oil adds a dash of heat and colour. The recipe is a delicious way to increase your intake of anti-inflammatory spices.

3 tbsp olive oil

1 onion, chopped

2 garlic cloves, crushed

2.5cm (1in) piece fresh root ginger, peeled and diced

4 large carrots, chopped

3 celery sticks, diced

500g (1lb 2oz) sweet potatoes, peeled and diced

600ml (1 pint) hot good-quality vegetable stock

200ml (7fl oz) coconut milk

2 tsp ground turmeric

1 tsp ground cumin

freshly grated nutmeg

salt and freshly ground black pepper

a handful of parsley, finely chopped

Chilli oil:

2 tbsp extra virgin olive oil

a good pinch of dried red chilli flakes

....

Variations:

• Substitute pumpkin for sweet potatoes.

• Add paprika (sweet or smoked) with the other spices.

• Serve the soup topped with some thinly sliced fried mushrooms.

1 Make the chilli oil: put the oil and chilli flakes in a small bowl and stir well. Set aside while you make the soup. The chilli will permeate the olive oil, turning it red and spicy.

2 Heat the olive oil in a large saucepan set over a low to medium heat. Cook the onion, garlic, ginger, carrots, celery and sweet potatoes for 10–15 minutes, stirring occasionally, until tender but not coloured.

3 Add the hot stock and bring to the boil. Reduce the heat immediately and simmer for 15 minutes, or until all the vegetables are cooked and have softened.

4 Blitz the soup in batches in a blender or food processor until it is thick, velvety and smooth. Return to the pan.

5 Stir in the milk and spices and reheat gently. If the soup is too thick for your liking, add some more milk to thin it to the desired consistency. Season to taste with salt and pepper, and stir in the parsley.

6 Ladle the soup into 4 shallow bowls and drizzle with the chilli oil. Serve piping hot.

SHAWARMA CHICKEN WRAPS

SERVES 4 | **PREP:** 15 minutes | **MARINATE:** 30 minutes | **COOK:** 20–25 minutes

Gluten-free wraps and tortillas are widely available in supermarkets, wholefood stores and delis. Choose free-range organic chicken, as it has more flavour and is healthier than mass-produced options.

500g (1lb 2oz) boneless skinned organic chicken breast fillets

400g (14oz) canned chickpeas, rinsed and drained

2 garlic cloves, crushed

3 tbsp olive oil

a squeeze of lemon juice

1 tsp cumin seeds, crushed

1 large aubergine, cubed

4 large gluten-free wraps

a handful of wild rocket

115g (4oz) dairy-free yogurt

harissa, to serve

Marinade:

1 tsp sumac

½ tsp ras el hanout

½ tsp ground turmeric

½ tsp ground cumin

½ tsp sweet paprika

a pinch of ground cinnamon

juice of ½ lemon

2 tbsp olive oil

2 garlic cloves, crushed

a handful of fresh mint, chopped

salt and freshly ground black pepper

....

Tip: Marinate the chicken a day in advance.

1 Make the marinade: dry-fry the ground spices in a frying pan for 1–2 minutes until they release their aroma. Do not let them colour. Tip into a large bowl and stir in the lemon juice, olive oil, garlic and herbs. Season. Add the chicken and stir until well coated. Marinate at room temperature for 30 minutes.

2 Meanwhile, coarsely mash the chickpeas with the garlic, 1 tablespoon olive oil, the lemon juice and cumin. Season to taste.

3 Heat the remaining olive oil in a ridged griddle pan over a medium to high heat. Add the aubergine and cook for 4–5 minutes, turning occasionally, until just tender and golden brown. Remove and drain on kitchen paper. Keep warm.

4 Add the chicken to the hot pan and cook for 10–15 minutes, until cooked. Remove and slice thinly.

5 Heat the wraps in the griddle pan. Spread the chickpeas and rocket over and place the aubergine and chicken on top. Add the yogurt and a drizzle of harissa, then roll up or fold over. Serve immediately.

ALMOND BUTTER CHICKEN PARCELS

SERVES 4 | **PREP:** 15 minutes

You can make these tasty parcels in minutes. Crisp iceberg lettuce leaves are the best ones to use as they are large enough to enclose the filling and do not go limp or tear easily, unlike most other lettuces. Miso paste is made from fermented soya beans and is rich in anti-inflammatory compounds.

85g (3oz) almond butter
2 tbsp miso paste
1 garlic clove, crushed
2-3 tbsp water
225g/8oz cooked chicken breast fillets, diced
a handful of coriander (cilantro), finely
  chopped
4 large crisp iceberg lettuce leaves
2 large carrots, coarsely grated
salt and freshly ground black pepper
balsamic vinegar or pomegranate
  molasses, for drizzling

....

Tip: This is a delicious way of using up leftover cooked chicken.

....

Variations:

- Add diced avocado, spring onions or baby plum tomatoes.
- For more crunch, include flaked or chopped toasted almonds.

1 Put the almond butter, miso, garlic and water in a large bowl and mix together well. If it's too thick, add some more water or some lemon or lime juice. Add the chicken and most of the coriander and stir gently until the chicken is coated.

2 Place the lettuce leaves on a clean work surface and divide the mixture between them. Top with the grated carrots and season lightly with salt and pepper.

3 Fold the sides of the lettuce leaves over the filling into the centre, and then fold the ends over, too, to make 4 neat parcels. Turn them over and place seam-side down on a plate. Serve immediately, drizzled with balsamic vinegar or pomegranate molasses.

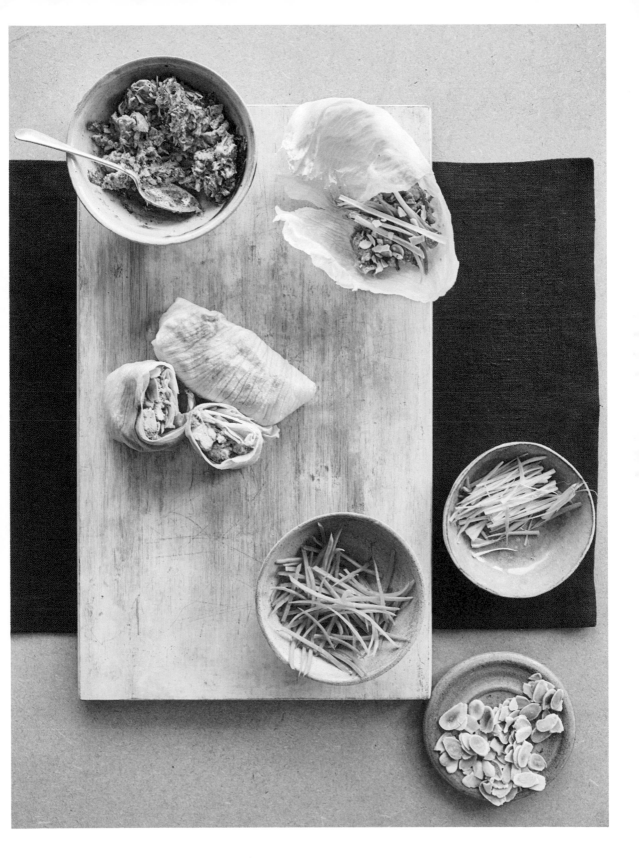

CHICKEN AND COCONUT CURRY

SERVES 4 | **PREP:** 15 minutes | **COOK:** 35 minutes

This delicately spiced curry served with nutty brown rice is a great way to get your daily anti-inflammatory ingredients and dietary fibre. If you want to make it hotter, add another chilli or a teaspoon of red chilli flakes.

3 tbsp olive oil

450g (1lb) skinned organic chicken breast fillets, cubed

1 red onion, thinly sliced

3 garlic cloves, crushed

1 hot red chilli, diced

2.5cm (1in) piece fresh root ginger, peeled and diced

1 tsp cumin seeds

2 tsp ground turmeric

1 tsp ground coriander

1 tsp garam masala

400ml (14fl oz) reduced-fat coconut milk

240ml (8fl oz) chicken stock

150g (5oz) fine green beans, trimmed and halved

200g (7oz) baby spinach leaves

100g (3½oz) dairy-free coconut yogurt

300g (10oz) brown rice (dry weight)

salt and freshly ground black pepper

Red onion relish:

1 red onion, diced

1 tsp garam masala

a small bunch of fresh coriander, chopped

a handful of fresh mint, chopped

juice of 1 lime

1 Make the relish: mix all the ingredients together and set aside.

2 Heat the oil in a deep frying pan set over a medium heat. Add the chicken and onion and cook, stirring, for 6–8 minutes until the onion is tender and the chicken is golden brown. Add the garlic, chilli, ginger and cumin seeds and cook for 2 minutes. Stir in the ground spices and cook for 2 minutes more.

3 Pour in the coconut milk and chicken stock and bring to the boil. Reduce the heat to low, cover the pan and simmer gently for 10 minutes. Add the green beans and cook for a further 5 minutes, until just tender. Stir in the spinach and cook for 2 minutes until it wilts. By this time the chicken should be cooked and the sauce will be creamy. Remove from the heat and stir in the yogurt. Season to taste.

4 Meanwhile, cook the rice according to the instructions on the packet.

5 Fluff up the rice and divide between 4 shallow serving bowls. Spoon the curry over the top and serve immediately with the relish.

YELLOW SPLIT PEA TARKA DHAL

SERVES 4 | **PREP:** 15 minutes | **COOK:** 50 minutes

When you're in need of comfort food, a bowl of spicy dhal is just the thing. Yellow split peas are high in fibre and, together with the ginger, turmeric, spinach, coconut and spices, have potent anti-inflammatory properties.

1 tbsp coconut oil

4 garlic cloves, crushed

1 tbsp grated fresh root ginger

1 red chilli, finely chopped

2 tsp black mustard seeds

2 tsp ground turmeric

2 cinnamon sticks

300g (10oz) yellow split peas, washed and drained

500ml (16fl oz) hot vegetable stock

1 x 400ml (14fl oz) can coconut milk

4 ripe tomatoes, roughly chopped

200g (7oz) baby spinach leaves

a handful of fresh coriander, chopped

juice of 1 lime

Tarka topping:

2 tbsp coconut oil

1 large onion, thinly sliced

1 tsp cumin seeds

4 green cardamom pods

4 whole cloves

1 red chilli, deseeded and thinly shredded

8 fresh curry leaves

....

Variations:

- Substitute red lentils for the yellow split peas.

1 Heat the coconut oil in a large heavy pan and cook the garlic, ginger and chilli over a low to medium heat for 2 minutes without colouring. Stir in the mustard seeds, turmeric and cinnamon. When the seeds start to pop, add the split peas, stock and coconut milk. Bring to the boil, then reduce the heat and simmer for 30 minutes.

2 Add the tomatoes and simmer for 15 minutes, or until the dhal is thick and creamy. If it's still a bit liquid, cook for a little longer; if it's too thick, add more stock.

3 Meanwhile, make the tarka topping: heat the oil in a frying pan over a medium heat and cook the onion, stirring, for 6–8 minutes, or until it starts to caramelize and turn golden brown. Add the cumin seeds, cardamom, cloves, chilli and curry leaves and cook for 2 minutes. Season lightly with salt and pepper.

4 Stir the spinach, coriander and lime juice into the dhal and when the spinach wilts, season to taste. Ladle into 4 shallow serving bowls and serve topped with the tarka.

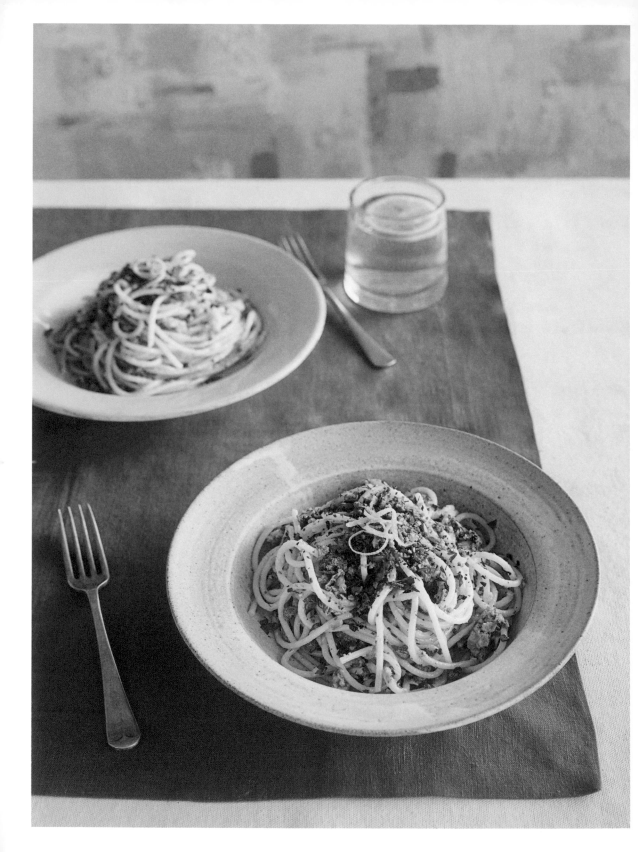

SPAGHETTI WITH SARDINES AND CAPERS

SERVES 4 | **PREP:** 5 minutes | **COOK:** 15–20 minutes

Using storecupboard ingredients makes this a quick healthy supper choice. Many types and brands of gluten-free pasta are available, including brown rice, millet, quinoa, buckwheat and mung bean.

75g (3oz) gluten-free fresh breadcrumbs
9 tbsp extra virgin olive oil
1 onion, diced
2 garlic clove, crushed
1 large juicy lemon
¼ tsp crushed red chilli flakes
3 x 125g (4½oz) cans sardines in olive oil, drained
5 tbsp capers, rinsed
400g (14oz) gluten-free spaghetti
a handful of fresh parsley, chopped
sea salt and freshly ground black pepper

....

Tip: Use the best-quality canned sardines you can find and, if wished, include some of the drained fishy olive oil in the pasta sauce.

....

Variations:
- Substitute chopped dill for the parsley.
- Sprinkle with some grated lemon zest just before serving.
- Add cooked chopped courgettes or green beans.

1 Fry the breadcrumbs in 3 tablespoons olive oil in a frying pan set over a low to medium heat, stirring occasionally, for 4–5 minutes or until golden brown. Remove and set aside.

2 Put the remaining oil in a large frying pan set over a low heat. Add the onion and garlic and cook for 6–8 minutes until tender and golden. Peel a long strip of lemon zest and add to the pan with the chillies, sardines and capers. Warm gently for 5 minutes, pressing down on the sardines to break them into smaller pieces. Remove the lemon strip.

3 Meanwhile, cook the spaghetti in lightly salted water according to the instructions on the packet.

4 Drain the spaghetti, reserving 240ml (8fl oz) tablespoons of the cooking water. Add the pasta to the oily sardine mixture, together with the lemon, juice and parsley. Add in the reserved water a little at a time until you have a smooth sauce. Toss well and season to taste.

5 Divide between 4 serving plates and top with the fried breadcrumbs. Serve immediately.

SALMON, COURGETTE AND ASPARAGUS LINGUINE

SERVES 4 | **PREP:** 10 minutes | **COOK:** 10 minutes

This speedy pasta dish is not only delicious but also gluten and dairy free. Always buy wild rather than farmed salmon if possible – it contains less saturated fat and a higher ratio of omega-3 to omega-6 fatty acids.

400g (14oz) gluten-free linguine (dry weight)
300g (10oz) thin asparagus, trimmed and halved
300g (10oz) skinned wild salmon fillet, cubed
fish stock (see below)
grated zest and juice of 1 small lemon
100g (3½oz) dairy-free yogurt
2 large courgettes, cut into ribbons with a potato peeler
a small bunch of fresh dill, chopped
salt and freshly ground black pepper

....

Tip: If you don't have fish stock, poach the salmon in water or a mixture of water and white wine.

....

Variations:

- Substitute smoked salmon for the fresh salmon fillets.
- Add trimmed and halved fine green beans or peas.
- Use chives instead of dill.
- Add diced red chilli or crushed chilli flakes.

1 Cook the linguine according to the instructions on the packet. Two minutes before the end of the recommended cooking time, add the asparagus to the pan. Drain well and return everything to the warm pan.

2 Meanwhile, put the salmon and enough stock to cover it in a pan and set over a low to medium heat. Simmer gently for 5 minutes, or until tender and cooked through. Remove with a slotted spoon and drain on kitchen paper. Pour away most of the stock and return the salmon to the pan with the lemon zest and juice. Season with salt and pepper and gently stir in the yogurt.

3 Add the creamy salmon mixture to the linguine together with the courgette ribbons and dill. Toss everything together gently to lightly coat the pasta strands.

4 Divide between 4 shallow serving bowls and serve immediately.

LEMON-CRUMBED GRILLED MACKEREL

SERVES 4 | **PREP:** 20 minutes | **COOK:** 5–6 minutes

The creamy texture of avocado in the guacamole complements the crispy breadcrumb topping on the fish and the added chillies contain powerful anti-inflammatory compounds called capsaicinoids.

85g (3oz) fresh gluten-free breadcrumbs
few sprigs of flat-leaf parsley, chopped
leaves stripped from a few thyme sprigs
grated zest and juice of 1 lemon
2 tbsp olive oil
8 mackerel fillets
salt and freshly ground black pepper
mixed salad leaves, such as rocket,
    watercress and baby spinach
gluten-free flatbreads or pita, to serve

Guacamole:

½ red onion, diced
1-2 fresh green chillies, diced
1 garlic clove, crushed
½ tsp sea salt crystals
juice of 1 lime
2 ripe avocados, halved, stoned, peeled
    and coarsely mashed
1 small bunch of fresh coriander, chopped
1 ripe tomato, deseeded and diced
freshly ground black pepper

1 Make the guacamole: crush the onion, chilli, garlic and salt in a pestle and mortar.

2 Mix the lime juice and mashed avocado in a bowl and stir in the coriander, tomato and crushed red onion mixture. Grind in some black pepper and set aside.

3 Preheat an overhead grill to high. In a bowl, mix together the breadcrumbs, herbs, lemon zest and juice, and olive oil.

4 Place the mackerel fillets, flesh-side up on a lightly oiled baking tray and spoon the breadcrumb mixture over the top of them.

5 Cook under the preheated grill for 5–6 minutes until the mackerel is cooked and the breadcrumbs are golden brown and crispy. Serve immediately with the guacamole, mixed salad leaves and warmed flatbreads or pita.

Tip: The guacamole can be prepared in advance and kept in the fridge until required.

Variations:
• Try red mullet, salmon or white fish.

CAULIFLOWER PIZZA

SERVES 4 | **PREP:** 20 minutes | **COOK:** 35 minutes

This delicious pizza is low in carbohydrates and gluten free. The base is made with cauliflower and it's so easy to prepare and cook. If wished, you can split the base mixture into two portions and make smaller pizzas.

1 large cauliflower (approx. 675g/1½lb)
115g (4oz) soft goats' cheese (or chevre)
1 garlic clove, crushed
a pinch of dried oregano
1 large organic free-range egg, beaten
salt and freshly ground black pepper
green pesto for drizzling
fresh basil leaves

Topping:
1 tsp olive oil
400g (14oz) canned chopped tomatoes
1 tbsp tomato paste
1 tsp sugar
a few sprigs of fresh basil, chopped
a splash of balsamic vinegar
100g (3½oz) soft goats' cheese
16 black olives, pitted

Tip: If you are dairy intolerant or vegan, substitute cashew cheese for the goats'.

Variations:
• Top the cooked pizza with fresh rocket and a drizzle of syrupy balsamic vinegar.
• Sweat onions in olive oil over a low heat, then stir in pine nuts. Spread over the tomato sauce before adding the topping.

1 Heat the oven to 200°C (180°C fan/400°F/Gas 6). Line a large baking sheet with parchment baking paper.

2 Discard the stem and leaves from the cauliflower, and separate the head into florets. Put them in a food processor and pulse until they have the consistency of crumbs. Transfer to a glass bowl, cover with cling film and microwave on high for 3-4 minutes. Spoon the cauliflower onto a stack of kitchen paper or a clean tea towel and press out any liquid until the grains are dry.

3 Mix the cauliflower in a large bowl with the goats' cheese, garlic, oregano, beaten egg and salt and pepper until it sticks together. If it's too dry, moisten with a little water or olive oil.

4 Place on the lined baking sheet and, using your hands, flatten and stretch the mixture until you have a large circle about 1.5cm (½in) thick. Bake in the preheated oven for 25–30 minutes or until crisp and golden brown.

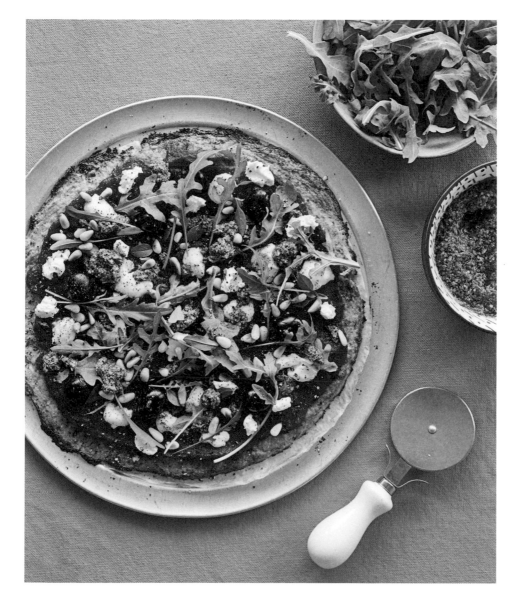

5 Meanwhile, make the topping: heat the oil in a frying pan set over a medium to high heat. Add the tomatoes, tomato paste, sugar and basil, and cook for 6–8 minutes until thick and reduced. Add the balsamic vinegar and salt and pepper to taste.

6 Spread the tomato sauce over the cooked pizza base and dot with goats' cheese and olives. Bake in the oven for 5–8 minutes.

7 Drizzle with pesto, add the fresh basil leaves, and serve immediately, cut into wedges.

STIR-FRIED CHICKEN WITH BROCCOLI

SERVES 4 | **PREP:** 10 minutes | **COOK:** 15–20 minutes

A true superfood, broccoli is a good source of fibre, plant protein and many nutrients, and this fast and fresh stir fry is a great way to increase your intake. The recipe is perfect for a quick, easy and healthy weeknight supper.

300g (10oz) brown rice (dry weight)

1 tbsp vegetable oil, such as flaxseed, walnut or avocado

500g (1lb 2oz) skinless organic chicken breast fillets, cut into thin strips

3 garlic cloves, thinly sliced

2.5cm (1in) piece fresh root ginger, peeled and grated

1 lemon grass stalks, peeled and thinly sliced

1 red chilli, thinly sliced

4 spring onions, thinly sliced

300g (10oz) tenderstem or purple sprouting broccoli, trimmed

grated zest and juice of 1 lime

2 tbsp tamari or gluten-free soy sauce

1 tsp toasted sesame seeds

4 tbsp toasted flaked almonds

1 Cook the rice according to the instructions on the packet.

2 Meanwhile, heat the oil in a wok or large deep frying pan set over a medium to high heat. Add the chicken and stir-fry briskly for 5 minutes until golden brown all over.

3 Add the garlic, ginger, lemon grass, chilli and spring onions and stir-fry for 2 minutes. Add the broccoli and cook for 2–3 minutes until it is just tender (al dente) but still retains its crispness. Stir in the lime zest and juice and tamari.

4 Serve immediately, sprinkled with the toasted sesame seeds and almonds, with the cooked rice.

....

Variations:

· Use calabrese broccoli (separated into small florets).

· Try adding shredded kale, spring greens or Savoy cabbage.

· Substitute the grated zest and juice of a small lemon for the lime.

GLUTEN-FREE COURGETTE NUT LOAF

SERVES 10–12 | **PREP:** 20 minutes | **COOK:** 1–1¼ hours

This delicious green-flecked loaf is made with oil instead of butter, making it dairy free as well as free from gluten and sugar. Depending on the flour you use, you may not need to add the xanthan gum. Check the ingredients on the packet and if it contains xanthan gum, don't add any more.

3 medium organic free-range eggs

2 tbsp powdered stevia

125ml (4fl oz) walnut or light olive oil, plus extra for brushing

300g (10oz) gluten-free flour

½ tsp xanthan gum (see above)

2 tsp gluten-free baking powder

½ tsp bicarbonate of soda

2 tsp ground ginger

1 tsp ground cinnamon

½ tsp ground nutmeg

½ tsp salt

3 large courgettes, grated

100g (3½oz) chopped walnuts

3 tbsp poppy seeds

Tip: Non-sugar sweeteners vary considerably. We have used 2 tbsp powdered stevia to replace 175g (6oz) sugar, but you should check a conversion chart for whatever plant-based sweetener you prefer to use.

Variations:

- Add a few drops of vanilla extract or some vanilla seeds scraped out of a pod.
- Vary the spices: try ground allspice or finely grated fresh root ginger.

1 Preheat the oven to 180°C (160°C fan/350°F/Gas 4). Lightly oil a 450g (1lb) loaf tin and line with baking parchment.

2 Beat the eggs, stevia and oil in a food mixer or processor until well blended. Mix in the flour, xanthan gum (if using), baking powder, bicarbonate of soda, spices and salt on a low speed. Add the courgettes and mix in gently with the walnuts and poppy seeds. If using a food processor, stir them in by hand.

3 Transfer the mixture to the prepared loaf tin and level the top. Bake in the preheated oven for 1–1¼ hours, or until the loaf is well risen and golden brown. Test if it's cooked by inserting a thin skewer into the centre – it should come out clean.

4 Leave the loaf to cool in the tin for 30 minutes before turning it out on to a wire rack. Leave until cold. Serve cut into slices.

5 Wrap the loaf in kitchen foil and store in an airtight container in a cool place for up to 3 days – longer in the fridge.

AVOCADO CHOCOLATE MOUSSE

SERVES 4 | **PREP:** 10 minutes | **COOK:** 4–5 minutes

A great way to sneak a vegetable into a dessert, the avocado gives this mousse a wonderful velvety texture. Avocados are among the most nutritious foods you can eat, rich in healthy fats as well as vitamins A, B3, B5, B6, B12, C, E and K, and essential minerals. They contain beneficial polyphenols and antioxidants that can protect against inflammation.

2 large ripe avocados

3 tbsp cocoa powder

a squeeze of lime juice

½ tsp vanilla extract

75g (3oz) coconut cream

100g (3½oz) plain dark chocolate
   (70% cocoa solids), broken into squares

5-10 drops liquid stevia or 60g (2oz)
   powdered sweetener, to sweeten

shaved dark chocolate and fresh
   raspberries, to serve

....

Variations:

• Sprinkle with coconut flakes.

• Top with blueberries and strawberries.

• Instead of vanilla extract, flavour the mousse with orange zest and juice.

1 Halve, stone and peel the avocados. Put the flesh in a food processor or blender with the cocoa powder, lime juice, vanilla extract and coconut cream. Blitz briefly until you have a smooth purée.

2 Melt the chocolate in a heatproof bowl suspended over a pan of gently simmering water. Remove the bowl from the heat and stir 1 tablespoon hot water into the chocolate. Let cool slightly.

3 Pour the melted chocolate into the avocado mixture and blitz until thoroughly mixed, smooth and creamy. Sweeten to taste with stevia and blitz again.

4 Spoon into 4 serving glasses or glass bowls and sprinkle with the chocolate shavings. Eat at room temperature or chill before serving. Serve with fresh raspberries.

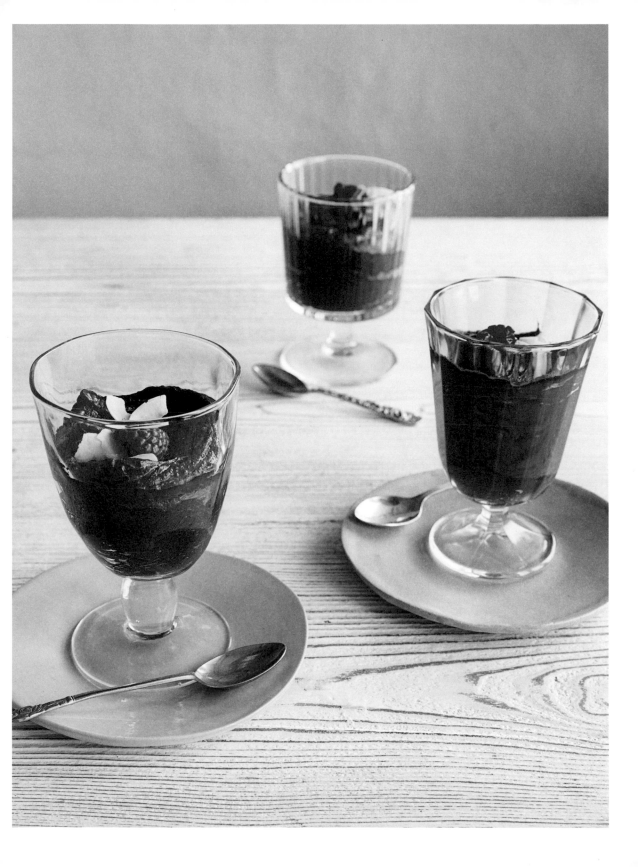

CHIA VANILLA SUMMER PUDDING

SERVES 4 | **PREP:** 10–15 minutes | **CHILL:** overnight

Make this delicious chia pudding in a glass bowl as below or divide between four individual screwtop glass jars before chilling. The chia seeds will swell overnight to thicken the mixture to a creamy tapioca-like consistency. The seeds are rich in protein and fibre, and provide a plant source of omega-3 fatty acids in the form of alpha linolenic acid (ALA).

600ml (1 pint) unsweetened almond milk or coconut milk

1 vanilla pod

½ tsp vanilla extract

liquid stevia, to taste

8 tbsp chia seeds

grated zest of 1 orange

4 tbsp dairy-free coconut yogurt

2 tbsp toasted coconut flakes

2 tbsp chopped almonds

300g (10oz) mixed berries, such as strawberries, raspberries, redcurrants, blueberries

1 Put the almond or coconut milk in a large bowl. Make a slit down the side of the vanilla pod and scape out the seeds into the milk. Add the vanilla extract, stevia, chia seeds and orange zest. Whisk well until everything is well combined and the chia seeds are distributed evenly throughout.

2 Cover the bowl with a lid or some cling film and leave to chill overnight in the fridge.

3 The following day, divide the thickened mixture between 4 serving bowls. Top each one with a spoonful of yogurt and sprinkle with the coconut and almonds. Top with the berries and serve.

Variations:

• Top with summer fruits, such as stoned cherries and sliced peaches.

• Sprinkle with toasted seeds, such as hemp, sunflower and pumpkin.

• Add a mashed banana to the milk and chia mixture before whisking and chilling.

BLUEBERRY OAT SQUARES

MAKES 9 squares | **PREP:** 15 minutes | **COOK:** 30 minutes

Eat these healthy fruity squares as a dessert with a spoonful of dairy-free yogurt or enjoy as a snack or teatime treat. They are high-fibre and free from gluten and refined sugar.

225g (8oz) rolled oats

2 tbsp chia seeds

1 tsp baking powder

2 large ripe bananas, mashed

1 large free-range organic egg, beaten

1 tsp vanilla extract

1 tsp liquid stevia

200g (7oz) blueberries

Variations:

- Substitute blackberries for the blueberries.
- Instead of vanilla, flavour with 1 teaspoon ground cinnamon.
- Vary the seeds: try flax or sunflower seeds.
- Add chopped almonds or walnuts to the oat mixture.

1 Preheat the oven to 180°C (160°C fan/350°F/Gas 4). Line a 20 x 20cm (8 x 8in) baking tin with baking parchment paper.

2 Place 50g (2oz) of the oats in a food processor or food chopper and blitz until finely ground. Transfer to a mixing bowl and stir in the remaining rolled oats, the chia seeds and baking powder. Add the mashed bananas, beaten egg, vanilla extract and stevia, and mix until well combined. If the mixture is a little dry, slacken with some almond milk; if it's too wet, add some more oats.

3 Put half of the mixture in the lined baking tin and spread it out evenly to cover the base. Spoon the blueberries over the top and then cover with the remaining oat mixture.

4 Bake in the preheated oven for 30 minutes or until cooked and golden brown. Remove and cool in the tin before cutting into squares. Store in the fridge in an airtight container for up to 5 days.

BIBLIOGRAPHY

THE SCIENCE:

1 Fowler, S.P., Williams, K., Resendez, R.G. 'Fueling the obesity epidemic? Artificially sweetened beverage use and long-term weight gain'. *Obesity* (2008). 16:8:1894–900.

LIFESTYLE:

1 Twohig-Bennett, C., Jones, A. 'The health benefits of the great outdoors: a systematic review and meta-analysis of greenspace exposure and health outcomes.' *Environmental Research* (2018).

2 Patel, A.V., Bernstein,, L., Deka, A., Spencer Feigelson, H., Campbell, P.T., Gapstur, S.M., Colditz, G.A., Thun, M.J. 'Leisure time spent sitting in relation to total mortality in a prospective cohort of US adults.' *American Journal of Epidemiology* (2010). 172:4:419–29.

NUTRITION:

1 Simopoulos, A.P. 'The importance of the ratio of omega-6/omega-3 essential fatty acids.' *Biomedicine and Pharmacotherapy* (2002). 56:8:365–79.

2 Czaja-Bulsa, G. 'Non coeliac gluten sensitivity – a new disease with gluten intolerance.' *Clinical Nutrition* (2015). 34:2:189–94.

3 Johnston, C.S., Kim, C.M., Buller, A.J. 'Vinegar improves insulin sensitivity to a high-carbohydrate meal in subjects with insulin resistance or type 2 diabetes.' *Diabetes Care* (2004). 27:1:281–82.

4 Prasad, S., Aggarwal, B.B. 'Turmeric, the golden spice.' *Herbal Medicine: Biomolecular and Clinical Aspects*, 2nd ed. (2011).

5 Lal, B., Kapoor, A.K., Asthana, O.P., Agrawal P.K., Prasad, R., Kumar, P., Srimal, R.C. 'Efficacy of curcumin in the management of chronic anterior uveitis.' *Phytotherapy Research* (1999). 13:4:318–22.

6 Takada, Y., Bhardwaj, A., Potdar, P., Aggarwal, B.B. 'Nonsteroidal anti-inflammatory agents differ in their ability to suppress NF-kappaB activation, inhibition of expression of cyclooxygenase-2 and cyclin D1, and abrogation of tumor cell proliferation.' *Oncogene* (2004). 23:57:9247–58.

7 Jurenka, J.S. 'Anti-inflammatory properties of curcumin, a major constituent of curcuma longa: a review of preclinical and clinical research.' *Alternative Medical Review* (2009). 14:3:277.

8 Hidaka, H., Ishiko, T., Furuhashi, T., Kamohara, H., et al. 'Curcumin inhibits interleukin 8 production and enhances interleukin 8 receptor expression on the cell surface: Impact on human pancreatic carcinoma cell growth by autocrine regulation.' *American Cancer Society* (2002). 95:6:1206–14.

9 Biswas, S.K., McClure, D., Jimenez, L.A., Megson, I.L., Rahman, I. 'Curcumin induces glutathione biosynthesis and inhibits NF-kB activation and interleukin-8 release in alveolar epithelial cells: Mechanism of free radical scavenging activity.' *Antioxidants and Redox Signaling* (2004). 7:1–2:32–41.

10 Hurley, L.L., Akinfiresoye, L., Nwulia, E., Kamiya, A., Kulkarni, A.A., Tizabi, Y. 'Antidepressant-like effects of curcumin in WKY rat model of depression is associated with an increase in hippocampal BDNF.' *Behavioural Brain Research* (2013). 239: 27–30.

11 Lien, H., Sun, W., Chen, Y., Kim, H., Hasler, W., Owyang, C. 'Effects of ginger on motion sickness and gastric slow-wave dysrhythmias induced by circular vection.' *American Journal of Physiology* (2003). 284:3:G481–9.

12 Lete, I., Allué, J. 'Effectiveness of ginger in the prevention of nausea and vomiting during pregnancy and chemotherapy.' *Integrative Medicine Insights* (2016). 11:11–17.

13 Halvorsen, B.L., Holte, K., Myhrstad, M.C.W., Barikmo, I., Hvattum, E., Fagertun, S., et al. 'A systematic screening of total antioxidants in dietary plants.' *Journal of Nutrition* (2002). 132:3:461–71.

14 Ahmed, R.S., Suke, S.G., Seth, V., Chakraborti, A., Tripathi, A.K., Basu, D.B. 'Protective effects of dietary ginger (zingiber officinales rosc.) on lindane-induced oxidative stress in rats.' *Phytotherapy Research* (2008). 22:7:902–6.

15 Kuriyama, S. 'Relation between green tea consumption and cardiovascular disease as evidenced by epidemiological studies.' *The Journal of Nutrition* (2008). 138:8:1548S–1553S.

16 Hursel, R., Viechtbauer, W., Westerterp-Plantenga, M.S. 'The effects of green tea on weight loss and weight maintenance: A meta-analysis.' *International Journal of Obesity* (2009). 33:956–61.

17 Tsartsou, E., Proutsos, N., Castanas, E., Kampa, M. 'Network meta-analysis of metabolic effects of olive oil in humans shows the importance of olive oil consumption with moderate polyphenol levels as part of the Mediterranean diet.' *Frontiers in Nutrition* (2019). 6:6.

18 Santangelo, C., Filesi, C., Varì, R., Scazzocchio, B., Filardi, T., et al. 'Consumption of extra-virgin olive oil rich in phenolic compounds improves metabolic control in patients with type 2 diabetes mellitus: a possible involvement of reduced levels of circulating visfatin.' *Journal of Endocrinological Investigation* (2016). 39:11:1295–1301.

19 Jurado-Ruiz, E., Álvarez-Amor, L., et al. 'Extra virgin olive oil diet intervention improves insulin resistance and islet performance in diet-induced diabetes in mice.' *Scientific Reports* (2019). 9:11311.

20 Esposito, K., Maiorino, M.I., Bellastella, G., Panagiotakos, D.B., Giugliano, D. 'Mediterranean diet for type 2 diabetes: cardiometabolic benefits'. *Endocrine* (2017). 56:1:27–32.

21 Salas-Salvadó, J., Bulló, M., Babio, N., Martínez-González, M., et al. 'Reduction in the incidence of type 2 diabetes with the Mediterranean diet: results of the PREDIMED-Reus nutrition intervention randomized trial.' *Diabetes Care* (2010). 34:1:14-19.

22 Beauchamp, G.K., Keast, R.S.J., Morel, D., Lin, J., Pika, J., et al. 'Ibuprofen-like activity in extra-virgin olive oil.' *Nature* (2005). 437:45–6.

23 Hjorth, E., Zhu, M., Cortés Toro, V., Vedin, I., et al. 'Omega-3 fatty acids enhance phagocytosis of Alzheimer's disease-related amyloid-ß42 by human microglia and decrease inflammatory markers.' *Journal of Alzheimer's Disease* (2013). 35:4:697–713.

24 Bosetti, C., Filomeno, M., Riso, P., Polesel, J., Levi, L., Talamini, R., Montella, M., Negri, E., Franceschi, S., La Vecchia, C. 'Cruciferous vegetables and cancer risk in a network of case-controlled studies.' *Annals of Oncolology* (2012). 23:8:2198–2203.

25 Su, X., Jiang, X., Meng, L., Dong, X., Shen, Y., Xin, Y. 'Anticancer activity of sulforaphane: the epigenetic mechanisms and the Nrf2 signaling pathway.' *Oxidative Medicine and Cellular Longevity* (2018).

26 Josling, P. 'Preventing the common cold with a garlic supplement: a double-blind placebo-controlled survey.' *Advances in Therapy* (2001). 18:4: 189–93.

27 Morihara, N., Nishihama, T., Ushijima, M., Ide, N., Takeda, H., Hayama, M. 'Garlic as an anti-fatigue agent.' *Molecular Nutrition and Food Research* (2007). 51:11:1329–34.

28 Różańska, D., Regulska-Ilow, B. 'The significance of anthocyanins in the prevention and treatment of type 2 diabetes.' *Advances in Clinical and Experimental Medicine* (2018). 27:1:135–42.

⌐WLEDGEMENTS

⌐y family, for always cheering me on and showing great enthusiasm for ⌐nank you to James, for your love, support and endless provisions of herbal ⌐⌐ to Lenny, precious creature, you were such therapy. Thank you to Jonathan, ⌐ng me to recover my own health, and for inspiring me to get into this field. Your care ⌐expert knowledge is a salve to many. I want to thank my publishing team, with special thanks to Victoria and Lisa; thank you for your support and encouragement throughout this process, and thank you to Heather, for the completely delicious recipes.

Anoushka Davy

PICTURE CREDITS

Adobe Stock: 14–15 **Shutterstock, Inc:** 4L, 8 Spectral-Design; 5L, 46 Jukov Studio; 6TL, 63 Fascinadora; 6TR, 45 Olimpik; 6MR, 51, 60 Oksana Mizina; 6BL, 59 New Africa; 6BR, 25 Andrey_Popov; 11 Designua; 17 SGr; 18 Fuss Sergey; 20 Musjaka; 49 tetxu; 55 PageSeven; 64 I Ketut Tamba Budiarsana; 68 Marian Weyo; 69 Photosiber **Unsplash:** 4R, 32 Blubel; 6ML, 37 Simon Migaj; 34 Jon Flobrant; 35 Yannic Laderach; 38 Julian Schultz; 41 David Mao; 61 Nathan Dumlao; 66 Anton Darius; 67 Matcha & Co; 70 Roberta Sorge; 73 Wouter Supardi Salari; 74 Monika Grabkowska; 77 Tijana Drndarski; 78 Katie Bernotsky; 80 Joseph Greve **Izy Hossack** © **Welbeck Non-Fiction Limited:** 5R, 84–121.

Senior Commissioning Editor: Victoria Marshallsay
Designer: Louise Evans
Photographer: Izy Hossack
Food and Props Stylist: Dominique Eloise Alexander
Copy Editor: Jane Birch
Proofreader: Anna Cheifetz
Indexer: Angie Hipkin
Production Controller: Gary Hayes